I believe the biological/nutritional approach
in this book shows clearly why the traditional
"professional" dietary community has been largely
ineffective in offering credible solutions to our
mounting problems of obesity, osteoporosis, diabetes,
etc. It is high time that we learn to cooperate with
our body chemistry instead of fighting with it. This
book provides a solid structure in which one may
accomplish this important shift toward a much
healthier and more reasonable, effective approach to
food and nutrition.

—Dion Boffo

Birchcreek client

In 1995 I had been diagnosed with a prediabetic
condition, but after my husband's sudden death,
my diabetes was rapidly becoming dangerously out
of control. I was gaining weight, my blood pressure
was rising, my asthma was getting worse, and
issues with my skin began to develop. During the
process to restore my health I preferred to—with
the total support and directions of my physician—
mix traditional medical care with alternative
solutions. After finding Birchcreek on the Internet, I
immediately felt optimism and excitement. Reading
about the Birchcreek method gave me hope. I decided
immediately that I would attend their retreat and
follow their recommendations. As soon as I arrived
in the Catskills, I felt the care and support from
everyone. The individual treatment, instruction, and
care made a huge and largely unexpected change in
my life. We not only received valuable information
about the biology of the body, breathing classes, and

exercise classes, but we also attended cooking classes and classes about food—and met many encouraging people. It was the practical piece I had been missing. I could do this!

With the help of the Birchcreek method my life has turned around, and my health started its recovery process within three weeks. I was able to establish my new Birchcreek lifestyle at home according to the given directions without any problem. With the continuing loving support of my therapist, physician, and friends, I continue my journey for building my "new" healthy productive life. Birchcreek has made it all possible.

—KATALIN FERENCZ-BIRO, PHD
BIOCHEMIST AND BIRCHCREEK CLIENT

This book is a timely solution to the growing problem of obesity. As we grapple with choosing an approach to health through nutrition and lifestyle changes, information can be confusing and conflicting. This book gives it to us straight and lays out a clear path to rapid and maintained weight loss. The advice is sound and foolproof with references that are tried and true. The only side effects to this weight-loss program are better health and more energy.

—MICHELLE FORGENIE
BUSINESS OWNER AND BIRCHCREEK ALUMNI

The Birchcreek Secret to Total Health will transcend your mind and transform your body. If you desire to attain the optimum level of health and effortlessly fight the "battle of the bulge," this brilliantly written book is a must-read. No more will you search for an answer to, "Which diet is best for me?" No more will you become discouraged going from diet to diet or doctor to doctor! The Odatos clearly state the most superior argument I have read for the need of mankind getting back to the "grassroots" of eating, back to the beginning before man invented prepackaged, frozen, denatured, and microwaved foods. They cut straight to the heart of the matter and, most importantly, provide the answer America needs to remedy the ever-burgeoning population of the chronically sick and morbidly obese. Throughout each page of this clever, entertaining, and educational book you will be challenged to think and be motivated to put what you learn into action. If you want to make a positive change…if you want to be empowered to live a life free from prescription drugs, excess pounds, and chronic disease, and do it with ease and enjoyment…don't pass up this opportunity to read *The Birchcreek Secret to Total Health*. Ron and Julie have helped thousands of people attain optimum health with the principles in this book, and I guarantee these principles *will* work for you!

—PATRICIA BINKLEY-CHILDRESS
PRESIDENT OF DESIGNS FOR FITNESS, LLC
AUTHOR OF *EDEN'S WAY,*
THE GARDEN'S PATH TO WELLNESS

We started the Birchcreek plan almost two years ago, and it was life changing. We are still on it, feeling great in body, soul, and spirit. Eliminating toxic foods and eating nutritionally, taking off weight, increasing mental alertness, and staying fit are all part of this wonderful plan from Birchcreek that Ron and Julie

Odato have taught us. By the way, their program is our lifestyle. It works! Read this wonderful book, and adopt it as your guide to total health!

—Larry and Judi Keefauver
Best-selling authors and
international speakers

The success of the Birchcreek system is truly exceptional. As I have been a guest of the program and worked in the behavioral and emotional wellness areas as a psychologist for many years, I have experienced firsthand the impressive results of the Birchcreek approach to weight loss and overall well-being. Its theoretical foundation and experiential application of behavior modification toward developing positive eating habits are sound and demonstrably effective.

—Rodrigo Villaseca, MA, LSCI

It is said that an apple a day keeps the doctor away! Apples contain vitamin C, which aid the immune system, and phenols, which reduce cholesterol. They also reduce tooth decay by cleaning one's teeth and killing off bacteria. Cornell University researchers have suggested that the quercetin found in apples protects brain cells against neurodegenerative disorders like Alzheimer's disease. The authors say in this book, "The evidence for nutritional therapy is becoming so strong that if doctors of today don't become nutritionists, then nutritionists will become the doctors of tomorrow." I truly believe that! Be encouraged; all your yesterdays have brought you to this book, and now all your tomorrows will be full

of living foods that bring health, energy, joy, and
long life!

—Nancy Engelhardt
Director, Catskill Mountain
Christian Academy

Ron and Julie Odato have written an explosive
book, and the truths they courageously put forth
contain the seeds of revolution! Not a revolution
of violence against a political, religious, or ethnic
issue, but a revolution of nutritional understanding
containing the power to restore wellness to millions
of decent people who are presently stuck in a cycle
of unsatisfying health and expensive drugs. Imagine a
stick of dynamite thrown into a snake pit, and prepare
to have your mind blown with good science, common
sense, and entertaining writing. Thanks, Ron and
Julie, for this important book…here's to your health!

—Bob Engelhardt
Pastor, radio personality,
and author of *White Like Snow*

THE
BIRCHCREEK
SECRET
TO TOTAL HEALTH

THE
BIRCHCREEK
SECRET
TO TOTAL HEALTH

RON AND JULIE ODATO

SILOAM

Most CHARISMA HOUSE BOOK GROUP products are available at special quantity discounts for bulk purchase for sales promotions, premiums, fund-raising, and educational needs. For details, write Charisma House Book Group, 600 Rinehart Road, Lake Mary, Florida 32746, or telephone (407) 333-0600.

THE BIRCHCREEK SECRET TO TOTAL HEALTH by Ron and Julie Odato
Published by Siloam
Charisma Media/Charisma House Book Group
600 Rinehart Road
Lake Mary, Florida 32746
www.charismahouse.com

Scripture quotations are from the New King James Version of the Bible. Copyright © 1979, 1980, 1982 by Thomas Nelson, Inc., publishers. Used by permission.

Cover design by Justin Evans
Design Director: Bill Johnson

Visit the author's website at www.weightlossretreat.com.

Library of Congress Cataloging-in-Publication Data:
Odato, Ron.
  The Birchcreek secret to total health / Ron and Julie Odato.
    p. cm.
  Includes bibliographical references.
  ISBN 978-1-61638-693-1 (trade paper) -- ISBN 978-1-61638-860-7 (e-book) 1. Weight loss--Psychological aspects. 2. Diet--Psychological aspects. 3. Nutrition--Psychological aspects. I. Odato, Julie. II. Title.
  RM222.2.O32 2012
  613.2'5--dc23
                                2012005862

This book contains the opinions and ideas of its author. It is solely for informational and educational purposes and should not be regarded as a

First edition

12 13 14 15 16 — 9 8 7 6 5 4 3 2 1

Printed in the United States of America

We dedicate this, our first book, to Pastor Robert and Nancy Engelhardt.

Besides our own parents, we have known very few who have sacrificed so much of their own time for our support and spiritual growth. Robert has consistently modeled humility, confidence, and strength, and Nancy is an example of what a godly woman should be. It was Nancy who prophetically suggested that Julie and I should start a business at Birchcreek that would help people with their health, which, in turn, has made this book possible.

CONTENTS

Contents

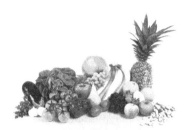

BIRCHCREEK'S COMMONSENSE
APPROACH TO DIET
AND LIFESTYLE

It is my privilege to write this foreword to Ron and Julie's new book about the healthy lifestyle promoted at Birchcreek Retreat. I am a sixty-three-year-old biochemist who works full-time as an executive in the pharmaceutical industry. My story is not unlike that of many others today. As we go through life, we experience unexpected and sometimes tragic changes that can affect our lives greatly. This was certainly true for me.

My husband's sudden, unexpected death in my arms left me completely in shock, overwhelmed, and feeling helpless. The EMS team had worked frantically to revive him, and as they transported him to the hospital, I rode by his side, emotionally frozen and shaken by fear. Sadly, the love of my life for twenty-seven years, my best friend and devoted husband, was gone.

I went home alone, walked into our home alone, and began to grieve alone. I kept thinking, "It's not supposed to be like this." I was overwhelmed, and I felt powerless. Although I was able to continue my full-time work, life as I had known it was gone forever. I thrust myself into my work, working late hours and neglecting to do the things that were necessary for my own well-being. As a result, my health deteriorated significantly.

In 1995 I had been diagnosed with a prediabetic condition, and now it was rapidly becoming dangerously out of control. I was gaining weight, my blood pressure was rising, my asthma was getting worse, and issues with my skin began to develop. Caught in a physical and emotional maelstrom, I was gradually being pulled into a very deep, dark place.

It was obvious to me that I needed to make significant changes in my life. I realized that continuing to keep myself in my own self-imposed lifestyle was self-abusive and did not honor or respect what my husband and I had both shared and valued. I had been lying down and letting life run over me. That was going to stop. I decided to get up, get out, and seize the life that was before me.

With my newfound resolve and with help and encourage-ment from my therapist, physician, and friends (coupled with the undying love of my husband in my heart), I began a process that would challenge me and bring me to the healthy, content, productive, and meaningful life that awaited me. I preferred to mix traditional medical care with alternative solutions, with the total support and directions of my personal physician. I attended two informative and useful health-related retreats. However, being able to apply what I had learned in a practical way proved difficult in my real world, where long hours and a demanding schedule were normal.

My background as a biochemist convinced me there must be a more natural way for me to control my health problems. I searched for a natural approach and a practical method that I could implement to validate my assumption.

I found Birchcreek Retreat on the Internet, and I started to feel optimistic and excited. Reading about the Birchcreek method gave me hope. Immediately I decided I would attend their retreat and follow their recommendations. As soon as I arrived in the Catskills, I felt the care and support from everyone. The individual treatment, instruction, and care made a huge and largely unexpected change in my life. I not only received valuable information about the biology of the body, along with breathing classes and exercise classes, but I also attended cooking classes and classes about food. And I met many encouraging people. It was the practical piece I had been missing. I could do this!

In table format below, I have summarized the positive health-related changes that I achieved during my three-week stay.

ATTRIBUTES	BEFORE BIRCHCREEK RETREAT	AFTER THREE WEEKS AT BIRCHCREEK RETREAT	NOTES
Birchcreek Method: No meat, no dairy, no processed food WEEK 1: Detoxification No solid food Juice 3x/day WEEKS 2–3: Juice 2x/day Raw salad for lunch Exercise: walking, breathing, weights, stretching	Organic, low-carbohydrate diet, according to glycemic index of food, including meat, cooked food, small amount of dairy No sugar, no white flour, no pasta, no cakes	After returning home, the Birchcreek method was continued.	Instructions were provided, and it was very easy to implement them.
Fasting blood sugar	200–240 mg/mL	130–140 mg/mL	Blood sugar measuring method: FreeStyle Lite Blood Glucose Monitoring System (Abbott)
Asthma	Wheezing; hard to breathe	No more wheezing; easy to breathe	No use of inhalers during and after Birchcreek

ATTRIBUTES	BEFORE BIRCHCREEK RETREAT	AFTER THREE WEEKS AT BIRCHCREEK RETREAT	NOTES
Hunger	Always hungry; could eat any time	No hunger; feel satisfied	
Craving	Craving for ice cream and sweets	No cravings	
General well-being	Occasionally tired, sad, and anxious	Clear-thinking, rather optimistic, goal-oriented, planning the future	

Within three weeks my life turned around, and my health started its recovery process. Without any problem I was able to establish my new Birchcreek lifestyle at home according to the directions that were given to me. With the continuing loving support of my therapist, physician, and friends, I continue my journey for building my new, healthy, productive life. Birchcreek has made it all possible.

Someone once said that it is not the number of times that you get knocked down; it is how many times you get up that makes the difference. If I could get up, so can you. Get up, get out, and get going…and go with the Birchcreek program!

—KATALIN FERENCZ-BIRO, MS, PhD

Authors' Note:

Birchcreek Retreat is a weight-loss and wellness center with two locations: the Catskill Mountains of New York state and in

Costa Rica. In this book we have collected what we teach in seminars and lead clients through in a hands-on program of restorative health and weight loss.

Because of the outstanding results, Birchcreek attracts people from around the world. One of those people was Katalin (Kati) Ferencz-Biro, MS, PhD, who stayed for a month at our retreat. She is a gracious and intelligent person whose lifelong career in biochemistry includes many accomplishments in the field of pharmaceutical drug development. Kati earned a master's degree in science and a PhD summa cum laude in biochemistry and chemistry from Eötvös Lóránd University in Budapest, Hungary. She has authored numerous scientific articles, particularly about research on interferon, which is used to treat cancer. She has international patents to her name and a well-established reputation in scientific research. Currently she is senior vice president of the Regulatory and Quality Assurance Departments at Hemispherx Biopharma in New Jersey.

Kati understands how the body was created to work as a chemical machine—one that needs proper nutrition to function to its full potential. The results Kati achieved at Birchcreek were a surprise to her, but they were no surprise to us, because her results are typical and anticipated at Birchcreek.

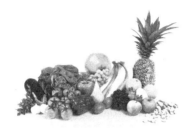

THE BIRCHCREEK GENESIS

In the late 1970s I (Ron) was hired as an engineer at Grumman Aerospace on Long Island, New York, and I began a continued course of education. While I was there, I won a couple of Project Sterling Awards, which are given for designs or innovations of new and improved methods or processes. I am proud to say that my intuitive ability to think out of the box rewarded me in that field.

After more than ten years in the aerospace industry, my wife and I opened a beautiful mountain retreat in the New York Catskill Mountains, located in the Forever Wild Forest Preserve. We operated a bed-and-breakfast in that setting for almost ten years, and my life spiraled downward into a sedentary lifestyle. I began to gain weight and began to age—ungracefully. Both Julie and I began to experience the same types of disorders that most people our age were experiencing. Our peers were no more or no less healthy than we were, and that's not saying much in America. A fifty-year-old person in America is not a picture of health any longer.

I began to look at poor health as a function of aging. But the more I read and studied, the more I discovered that today's new science concerning health and well-being puts a tremendous emphasis on diet and lifestyle. I began to learn that a person's body heals from within. It is not the use of a Band-Aid or a cast on an arm or a medication that heals a problem. The body heals itself because it is designed to do so if given the opportunity. I became so excited that I began to invest myself in studying about nutrition, learning all I could about it, practicing it myself, attaining certification on the whole subject, and finally telling other people about it. How wonderful it was for me to closely monitor and see each of my ailments disappear, month by month, until they were gone!

For me, regaining my health through good nutrition was a miracle. Julie and I turned our B and B into a retreat center. Now, as the director of the Birchcreek Weight Loss and Wellness Retreat, I am a man who has added years of health and vitality to my life. I am sixty-three years old, and I feel better than I have since I was in my thirties. This is true because of the life change that I made more than ten years ago. The change I decided to make for the sake of my own well-being was prompted by the experience of watching both my parents and my wife's mom die of cancer.

Big Changes

Having reached an age where things were beginning to go wrong in our own health, Julie and I decided to get healthy. Instead of looking only at traditional vitamins, supplements, and a kind of diet that most people who appeared to be healthy were eating, I wanted to go over the top and do things right.

I found out about a diet and a style of eating that was foreign to me, and within six months I had completely changed my dietary habits and lifestyle. The results of this way of eating restored my health and enabled rapid, aggressive weight loss. I had never felt better in my life than I did during that transition, and now, almost eleven years later, I still feel completely healthy, strong, and energized.

Not only do I have a story to tell, but I also have a business that represents that story and that is helping people do the same thing I did. The testimonies and the life-changing experiences that I have witnessed during what we call the "Birchcreek Jump-Start Your Life Program" are nothing short of miraculous.

People have watched as my life turned around. I was a person who seemed to be on his way to heart disease or worse. Transformation to a picture of health came almost overnight. Naturally people wanted to know what my wife and I had done. They could hardly believe it when we offered them the solution to what we thought was hurting us. Probably the most difficult thing for people to accept and comprehend was that, even in our highly technological world, what had turned out to transform our health and appearance was simply changing the food we ate and adopting an active lifestyle. Now for us it has become natural.

Some people we shared with tended to believe that it might play a part in the solution, while some thought it just might be that wonderful answer they were seeking. Others just dismissed it because it sounded too easy. In our society, as a matter of fact, we have been taught that if it sounds too good to be true, it probably isn't. In this case it is too good and it *is* true.

For years now we have been helping other people change their lifestyles so they can experience what we have experienced. It is not a matter of telling them what to eat or what not to eat. That would only give them a prescription for failure. Instead we have developed the ways and means of getting to that final goal, and we have perfected a program that works for everyone.

Commercials and advertisements promise us all the results and all the satisfaction from all the products they are trying to sell. The result is distraction and confusion. We experiment with these products because we don't know what is really true. We are confused because perhaps we have never heard the truth. Nothing really sounds right, so we grasp at anything, hoping that it may be the true solution. Our natural tendency is to grasp at something we think we can achieve, perhaps the quickest or easiest or the least difficult of all the choices we have at our disposal. We reach for that silver bullet. This person is selling this product or service, and he says that it cures a multitude of ills, and more.

Many people come to us with serious disorders. Many come just because they want to lose stubborn weight. Everyone goes away excited and vastly improved! Why? At Birchcreek they experienced something they didn't anticipate ever happening to them, and it represents real, measurable improvement. The truth is, we have found the only way to improve health, to sustain a healthy weight and vitality, to roll years off your appearance, and to add years to life. It is simply to change what you eat.

HOW WE GOT HERE

In order to realize where Birchcreek is today, we need to travel back to that point in time when Julie and I began to seriously question the role medicine and science have played on the American scene. We were discouraged seeing friends and family succumb to the same diseases mankind has always fallen to without much improvement to their life expectancy or quality of life.

When my parents and Julie's mom passed away, we felt that the world ended. Any hope to avoid these kinds of fatal maladies evaporated before our eyes. Our loved ones, who just a short time ago had been living apparently healthy lives filled with vitality, had all died from cancer. Cancer is just one of many, many diseases that is life threatening, and we have learned to consider it normal to suffer later in life from one disease or another. Although I had believed in my youth that disease would not happen to me, the possibility became a stark reality when the people around me, with whom I had grown up and whom I considered ageless, succumbed to disease.

We have all known people who develop these "difficult-to-overcome" diseases, and we have heard them promise in the early stages, "I'm going to devote myself to beating this thing." Lo and behold, before long the fabric not only of their resolve and confidence but also the resolve and confidence of everyone around them begins to wilt as the disease takes its toll. Before long it becomes natural for friends and family to accept the poor state of health of their loved one and to accept the inevitability of their imminent death. No longer are these people thought of or remembered as the vital people that we knew just a short time ago, but rather they are considered "sick" people.

Does this have to be commonplace? The fact that some people do overcome these diseases and that their resolve and courageous confidence do succeed gives us hope. But what made the difference? Is it their courage, confidence, and resolve? Those qualities do play a part in recovery. Or is it more? Is it that, from the point of view of genetics and body chemistry, the people who overcome these things have an advantage over those who succumb to disease? We are built differently, and some of us are more susceptible to things.

Even a diagnosis can take the life out of a person. In the cases where people believe that they cannot succeed in overcoming a life-threatening illness, not only is their resolve drained, but also their immune systems have been damaged without recourse. Already their physiology is in compromised condition, and the treatments offered knock them for a loop. Once diagnosed with a serious, life-threatening disease, some people have nothing left working for them. Forget weight loss or improved diet. Often these people say, "The therapy is so uncomfortable, I don't want to go through it any more. Just leave me alone." In their minds failure is inevitable, so giving up is normal. Well, it is not inevitable, and it is not normal.

AVERAGE IS NOT NORMAL

We may be scared by the averages we continually read about. Staggering numbers of people seem to be developing heart disease, cancers, diabetes, and all the other debilitating diseases. Osteoporosis and neurological disorders such as Parkinson's disease and Alzheimer's disease are rising too, although they may seem statistically less threatening. Is this the "new normal"? By no means. We should never cross-pollinate the statistical averages with our own life experiences. Average is not normal. I repeat this statement often! It is *not normal* for people to get heart disease, cancer, diabetes, and osteoporosis. Normal people don't get those diseases. These abnormal conditions develop from a lifetime of eating an inappropriate diet.

The food you eat can restore health and vitality, sometimes almost overnight. I learned when I was young enough to care how I looked—and when I turned fifty—I looked horrible. I looked as if I was carrying around bricks. People noticed my appearance, and that bothered me. Then I discovered that the diet that would make me healthy would make me shed pounds more rapidly than I had ever experienced! In one week people recognized the difference. Not only did my physical appearance change and improve, but also so did my temperament and my frame of mind. I was flying high.

By following the advice in this book, you will see changes in yourself, and they will be the catalyst to move you forward. You will watch your physiology change right before your very eyes. People will notice that you seem happier. You will find yourself thinking more clearly. No longer will your problems appear as mountains to you. When you're feeling better because you have adopted a new nutritional lifestyle, those mountains will return to being the molehills they should be.

Physiologically you will find improvement on every level: in your appearance, behind the scenes in your nervous system, in the function of your organs, and in the production and distribution of hormones. As everything begins to work right, that incredible, miraculous body you have will begin to do what it was designed to do. Your body was designed to resist breakage, and it was designed to resist disease and debilitation.

My goal for this book is that you, the reader, will know that there is hope and that you will gain confidence in your own body's ability to restore health and vitality with the help of a diet that was perfectly designed for you. I also hope that this way of life becomes the norm and that we can all turn the corner, both in the science of medicine and in the hearts and minds of people who rely so heavily on medicine. Enough of the poor results from the growing tsunami of illnesses that have overtaken us for the past fifty years. My wife and I hope that the program we have designed will be useful to you, regardless of your age, health status, ailments, or weight. No matter how despondent you may have become from whatever diagnosis you've been given, and no matter how many times your diet has failed, this time can be different. You can allow your body to do the work. The results will amaze you.

YOU CAN'T BUY HEALTH

You know the expression, "You can't buy health." When your health is gone, you lose the ability to plan your future or to appreciate this incredible adventure called life. It is true that you can't buy your health, but too many of us spend most of our lives purchasing and eating the very foods that earn us sickness and disease. The candy bars, the soft drinks, the fried foods, and our overreliance on meat and dairy products have served us poorly. Yet we think that these foods are adequate. If the whole purpose of food was to store fat and make us uncomfortably lethargic, then these foods would be at the head of the class!

Our bodies are wondrous machines designed for longevity and health, plus vitality into old age. What makes a human being unique is our makeup of body, mind, and spirit. No other creature on earth has all three components. And that's why we can have hope. Equipped with these very special, distinctly human qualities, behavioral instincts can be left behind. Human beings work on a higher order and have been designed for a better purpose than the other animals. We can draw upon our reason, intellect, and free will to make healthy choices that improve and prolong our lives. Now we often make very poor choices that are not conducive to our well-being. But we can learn and make changes.

Not only do we have the ability to control and alter our own environment, but also we are the only creatures on earth that can explore new ways of approaching things. With that kind of latitude imbedded in our intelligence, we naturally explore the realm of food and nutrition. The expression "necessity is the mother of invention" pertains only to humans. In life-and-death situations, animals have no way of improvising alternatives or deciding to adapt to changes. When their environment suffers a radical change, they perish.

When a human being's environment changes radically, that person will explore and improvise until solutions can be found. People will alter their environments to suit their comfort as much as possible. They will adjust their food to suit their tastes.

Our intelligence drives us to seek satisfaction in every area of life, but we don't often do a good job of it. Unchecked by consequences, we determine to make our world more comfortable for ourselves, which includes enjoying the pleasure of food without understanding its nutrition. Why do we indulge in such unnatural choices? We do it because we can. It is not only the way we eat but also the way we dress, what we do to our bodies, the way we think, and the activities we indulge in. The consequences of our choices show up years later when things begin to break, deteriorate, and disintegrate.

CONVENIENCE AND TASTE

Here we are, thinking ourselves smarter than ever, having engineered our world far away from the way it should be. When it comes to food, convenience and taste drive us like lemmings over a cliff without consideration for our own well-being. Busy Americans consider free time a premium. Taking time to prepare meals is a thing of the past for most modern families. Always on the go, we prepare food oftentimes by "adding water." As a society we have lost or forgotten the wisdom of the past, and we have no desire to emulate our parents in any way.

Our food tastes have been reengineered. No longer satisfied with the natural taste of natural, we've reached a point where our threshold of taste isn't satisfied until we have fully reached the extreme limits of our likes and dislikes. The fast-food companies in America, well known for their engineering of tastes through the manufacture of foods that stimulate both thirst and hunger, continue to "improve" the size of their packaging and their presentation propaganda.

We may be the smartest society in history, yet we are also one of the most unhealthy and sick ones. The fact is, we are lost, although we do not realize it. We look for the latest data or some new solution to our problems. We don't need a doctor's evaluation to inform us that our joints ache, we lack energy, and we are so physically challenged that climbing just one flight of stairs leaves us breathless, with hearts beating wildly. What do we do when we begin to realize something might be wrong? We go to the doctor, hoping to receive some advice or a medicine that can heal us or at least reduce or eliminate our discomfort.

There is another way! You can discover the facts and the simple truths of good nutrition. Scores of people from around the world have done so over the past decade, and you can too. Go back to Genesis. Step into health. Make good choices for yourself based on truth. Stop being driven by your cravings and desires. The Birchcreek program is for you; read on and take it to heart!

CHAPTER 1

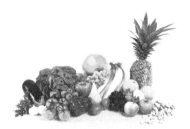

NEVER AGAIN COUNT CALORIES, CARBOHYDRATES, PROTEIN, OR OUNCES

Never again count calories, carbohydrates, or protein or weigh your food. Eat as much as you like, not as much as can fit, and feel complete. Eliminate cravings, bingeing, and that ferocious sweet tooth. Finally begin to lose weight rapidly and consistently; regain and maintain not only a youthful appearance but also your health—long into old age. It is so simple anyone can do it! How? Start by reading this book and reeducating your biology to do for you what it does best.

The information in this book is not readily found. You won't actually trip over it. Yet it requires little validation. In tens of thousands of people who benefit from the results, a simple dietary lifestyle change delivers success. Science and medicine have often failed to create a place of importance for natural healing through a restorative, plant-based diet, because research is embedded in the institutional dictatorship of the pharmaceutical industry. Nevertheless, more and more people are finding their way to this remarkably easy approach to rapid, healthy weight loss and health restoration.

It is not the responsibility of the general public to become educated in science and medicine in order to live a healthy lifestyle. But lifestyles of the twenty-first century are so foreign to human biology that we harm ourselves on a daily basis. Our lifestyles only remotely resemble anything of the natural way in which every other creature on earth lives, from the air we breathe to the water we drink and the foods we eat, along with our lack of physical exercise. Even our own special place in the animal kingdom has been so distorted that our human nature has been strained to the breaking point.

We have asked our species to cope with so much more than our genetics can embrace—and it shows. Our bodies require consistency of proper nutrition, something all creatures require to maintain order. When this order is obstructed, it is not a stalemate we encounter. No, what follows are the diseases and maladies we suffer today. And the opposite is equally true. Return to the nourishment of living foods and witness the body's remarkable ability to restore and maintain health and vitality. It is easier than you might think.

What if I told you that losing weight and staying healthy are less about too many calories and more about regulating proper chemistry? Rather than focusing this book on nutrition, which can be dry and boring, this book offers understanding. You will learn *why* you are obese and sick and how to correct these conditions for good. As science gets demystified, you will be entertained with simple, clear, logical, and effective explanations.

With the knowledge of how your body responds to good, healthful foods as well as its lack of tolerance for dangerous foods, you will be able to negotiate a new diet and lifestyle. Your results will include rapid, healthy weight loss, a continually detoxifying body, and restoration of health and vitality long into old age. And the best part is... you don't have to sacrifice taste or your love of food.

As you read this book, consider those immortal truths that need no validation but indeed need reintroduction. The relationship between our health and what we eat is not new information—but we have lost track of it.

ANCIENT WISDOM

Long before the development of modern pharmacology (in the 1800s), the forefather of medicine, Hippocrates, coined the creed for contemporary nutritional philosophy: "Let the food be thy medicine and medicine be thy food."

And long before Leonardo da Vinci autopsied his first cadaver and began to understand the human digestive tract, the Scriptures identified the way we were created to eat: "And God said, 'See, I have given you every herb that yields seed which is on the face of all the earth, and every tree whose fruit yields seed; to you it shall be for food'" (Genesis 1:29).

So how can we get back to Genesis? Humans could not have known in the ancient times of the Bible that this scripture was to become the foundation of modern twenty-first-century nutritional science. Four thousand years before the first digestive enzyme was discovered, biblical wisdom and sages revealed the foods from which we could obtain the most beneficial nutrition.

Nutrition has overtaken the unfolding science of biochemistry and genetic engineering with obvious results that can hardly be disputed. You can easily log on to a computer and ask any question about a plant-based diet or what part it plays in health and longevity, and your results will undoubtedly lead you to one of two camps.

The approach of traditional medicine for the most part resists giving diet and nutrition a major emphasis. Part of the reason is to protect both scientific turf and an enormous financial empire. Alternatively the second camp demonstrates rather conclusively the power and effectiveness of plant-based diets and offers ongoing education to anyone who desires to pursue it.

Our accomplishments at Birchcreek result from adhering to the propositions proved by the most recent science, which lines up with the ancient wisdom. Every day we see how the human body responds almost immediately to a change from a diet of mostly meat; dairy; and fried, processed, and cooked foods to that of a diversified plant-based diet. By fueling the human body with nutrition in its most beneficial forms, we see quick and positive results.

Food and nutrition are indeed in the midst of a medical revolution. In fact, it is nutritional science that is delivering the latest deathblow to the old, preposterous idea that without science and medicine we cannot hope to live long and maintain health.

Nutritional science, not medicine or the dictates of pharmaceutical companies, now stirs up the latest controversy over how and what we should be eating as *Homo sapiens*. The medical industry resorts to prescribing an infinite number of pharmaceuticals, expensive treatments, and unnecessary testing, while malpractice, misdiagnoses, and lawsuits proliferate.

The economy of sickness creates much wealth. In fact, in our disgracefully obese culture we have to lay some of the blame for the declining health of Americans directly at the feet of medical science, paired as it is with commerce. At last we are seeing increasing exposure in the media about the dangers of consuming a meat and dairy diet. This previously unfamiliar subject is becoming much better understood, as confirmed by the array of websites, studies, and scientific findings.

More progressive hospitals now promote and offer plant-based cleansing/detoxifying and high-nutrition diets to seriously ill patients. These purposeful treatments enhance every aspect of recovery from illness. Wouldn't it be wonderful to find the personal assurance that we never have to suffer a dire diagnosis of illness in the first place—simply because of following proper nutrition all along? The more people realize the truth about nutrition, the more the sound of truth will become deafening—as it echoes in the halls of empty hospitals and clinics.

LIVING FOODS

As thousands are taking advantage of this radically natural approach to rapid, healthy weight loss, renewed vitality, and health restoration, the medical community is at long last waking up to the abundance of case studies that are beginning to document the positive results of a plant-based diet. How can we change from a reliance on a diet of meat, dairy, and mostly cooked, fried, and nuked foods to a diet of mostly "living foods"? What are "living foods"?

Living foods are the kinds of foods every animal on the face of the earth consumes. And in consuming them, most of the natural animal kingdom avoids the wholesale disease and maladies that befall mankind.

What if we followed the leading edge of research studies about how much plant-based diets can do? I heard one of the nutritional giants say, "The evidence for nutritional therapy is becoming so strong that if doctors of today don't become nutritionists, then nutritionists will become the doctors of tomorrow." In the past twenty years a virtual revolution in science and medicine has tilted the path to health and longevity from medicine and pharmaceuticals to the power of the properly nourished human body to maintain and restore health and vitality. The path to optimum health is being redefined as I write. With the power of biochemistry, we are now capable of following the path of the metabolic transfer of nutrition from food to the release of energy within every human cell.

But how can Americans know how to eat and what to eat when there are so many diets from which to choose? Unfortunately the obvious truth about what we should eat has been dictated by how much change can be accepted by the general population. What quality-providing changes will industries implement, and at what cost? So the public is allowed to consume only bite-sized hints of the solution. And in fine print, which provides far less than the important fanfare it deserves, we see and hear, "Eat more fruits and vegetables; eat less meat and dairy."

FAD DIETS

New fad diets are often driven by taste appeal rather than nutritional needs, and by the well-entrenched notion that the American diet must include a large percentage of meat. In reaction fad diets multiply annually. The Atkins diet is an example of a recent fad diet. What could be more unnatural than the Atkins diet? The diet eliminated fruits, along with complex and whole-grain carbohydrates. Atkins created an uproar by announcing the opposite of what recent scientific findings were beginning to tell us. Talk about confusing! Consume nothing but bacon, eggs, steak, pork, and chicken while eliminating plant-based carbohydrates—it sounded ridiculous, but initially people got results. And what were the results? Along with rapid weight loss, continuing on this regimen for a long period of time came at the expense of loss of organ health. The latest findings have created the necessary course correction for this once total animal protein diet. Sadly, the maintenance program that was birthed out of necessity for the Atkins diet looks very similar to the "balanced" standard American diet. And look where that has taken us!

There is also the blood-type diet, in which your ideal food choices are based on whether your blood is type A, B, AB, or O. As a whole, neither this diet nor any of these fad diets have shattered any records, nor have they resulted in any measurable long-term major health benefits. All of them will work if all you want to do is lose weight. Weight loss is not the whole issue. I could endorse a candy bar diet that will help in weight loss! But is that useful or a healthy choice for long-term well-being and vitality?

I could give pages to other fad diets. You have heard of most of them. The bottom line here is the fact that we are allowing ourselves to be persuaded to fuel ourselves improperly. The foods we are eating are putting such a burden on our systems that we are sicker and fatter than ever. Our biological operating systems were not designed for such burdens. If it weren't for advances in medicine, we would be dying of heart disease and diabetes at an even more alarming rate. Oh that's right; we are dying from heart disease, cancers, diabetes, and a host of other ailments at an alarming rate—medicated as we go. The mortality statistics of a hundred years ago have been shattered. For the most part we have beaten TB, polio, wholesale death from influenza, infant mortality, and women dying in childbirth. That's the good news. But considering our present twenty-first-century diet, if we had not developed prescription drugs and medical interventions, our life expectancy might not have increased at all.

THE POWER OF INFORMATION

Genetic science and biochemistry have opened up even more complex relationships between health, illness, and the foods we consume. The "new kid on the block" is new understandings about sensitivities to grain foods. In some scientific circles it is believed that our recent six- to ten-thousand-year relationship with agriculture and systematic farming, by which we have become dependent upon gluten-rich grain products, may be the root cause of some serious digestive diseases and cancers. This information could very well cause us great confusion about what to eat. If grains are now labeled dangerous, and yet grains have been proven to be such an essential part of a healthy diet, we need a context in which to understand and apply this information.

Then we have the new and explosive evidence concerning the power and health benefits of ample doses of vitamin D_3, with deficiency in D_3 apparently lying at the heart of many deleterious health conditions. The evidence is so new, so alarming, and so scientifically sound. When added to what we already know to be true, this new information can yield even more positive effects with a plant-based diet. Birchcreek is preparing a supplemental booklet on this subject.

The Birchcreek program does not promote extremes. Understanding why a certain food type may be more harmful than good is vitally important. A person can be tested for sensitivity to gluten in grain foods. New tests are far more refined than in the past and offer us the privilege of identifying these sensitivities. Sensitivity to certain foods does not condemn that food to a guilty-as-charged verdict. At Birchcreek we have witnessed the most severe allergies and food sensitivities dramatically reduced or completely eliminated with our program. Often, a complete resumption of consuming the very foods to which an individual was so allergic in the past can be realized.

We recognize that it is not necessarily that we happen to have an allergic reaction when we eat a certain food, but rather that we have become sensitized through a diet that has left our overworked and underpaid immune systems reactive and sensitive. Our bodies suffer ever-growing deficiencies and toxicities from foods we were not designed to eat in the first place. The poor and dangerous foods we insist on eating as Americans have turned out to be the culprits that have started us down a path of deficiency, toxicity, sensitivity, and, ultimately, incompatibility with certain foods.

Grains and other complex carbohydrates contain important fiber that binds to sugar. These complex carbohydrates require mastication (chewing) and the introduction of an enzyme called amylase to begin the release of this sugar into the bloodstream. This is a well-designed, slow process that offers long release of energy and a regulated release of insulin, a hormone. Insulin transports the sugar (glucose) into the cells where sugar (glucose) is utilized as cellular energy. The human intestinal tract aids this process by separating the fiber from the rest of the nutrition. Once in the bloodstream, glucose can be absorbed and utilized by the body. Grains are the perfect nutrition food because they complete the slow cycle of feeding all the cells of the body.

And by eating a wide variety of plant food, one is less likely to be deficient in essential nutrients. The readily available nutrition in whole foods such as fruits, vegetables, grains, legumes, seeds, nuts, herbs, and spices offer the essential vitamins, minerals, bioflavonoids, and essential fatty acids necessary for proper biological function.

So where do we go from here? Follow Julie and me through this most fascinating story that has led to successful change in our health, appearance, and lives. We changed from very overweight proprietors of a well-known bed-and-breakfast where we served bacon, eggs, muffins, sausage, French toast, breads, and quiches, to the founders of Birchcreek Weight Loss and Wellness Retreat. We have not only dramatically improved our own lives but also the lives of thousands of others through our carefully designed and well-tested program.

CHAPTER 2

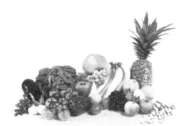

WHAT'S YOUR FRAME OF
REFERENCE FOR FOOD?

Your frame of reference is your model of understanding, what you believe to be true. What is your frame of reference in regard to food? I will warn you, this question is loaded. Your understanding of the role food plays in your life will range from addiction to unimportant necessity. I feel safe in saying that most Americans are lost and confused when it comes to eating properly. Just the word *properly* means different things to different people and is therefore a relative term. In spite of (or because of) your personal relationship with food, you may be aware of a need to alter your eating habits. The latest buzz concerning weight loss may have persuaded you to make changes, and you know your health can be affected by the foods you eat.

For most Americans a course correction seems more like a shot in the dark than a dependable solution. Too often, when we decide on a new diet, we choose convenience rather than correctness. We are lost in a sea of confusing and hard-to-understand reasons for preferring one diet to another. How can we find our way back home? Confronted with a maze of food choices, with all sorts of dietary information coming our way, how do we choose?

Think about finding your way home if you were truly lost. Imagine if someone put a blindfold on you and drove you a long distance, then put you on an airplane and flew you another long distance, and then put you back in an automobile and dropped you off in the middle of a forest. When the blindfolds are removed, you are lost. Unless you are highly specialized in field survival, you have no true frame of reference, and you can't possibly know where you are. You need to know roughly where you are in order to begin your journey home.

In today's world, unless you have an education in nutrition, you can find yourself just as lost when it comes to correcting your diet and lifestyle. You are not alone; this is a relatively accurate description of where most Americans find themselves.

When we hear "Eat more fruits and vegetables, less meat and dairy" and "Exercise for health," we pick up a degree of perspective of the solution. However, even if such slogans gave a complete solution, we would probably only adopt the ones that provide for our comfort and suit our taste. Besides, we will pick only the ones we think we can do.

It's a gamble. We can only hope that this diet or that exercise program has the solution to our problem. Most people really don't know enough about the science behind the claims of a particular diet or exercise program to make an educated choice. Often these choices contain only part of the solution. Most diets omit sustainable nutrition. And exercise programs turn out to be created more for the masses than for the needs of the individual.

You need to adopt a plan that covers all the bases, a plan without shortcuts. And you cannot make an intelligent choice without knowledge and understanding. Only with facts and an understanding of those facts can you ever hope to make wise decisions. Equipped with knowledge and understanding, you can not only make good choices and implement wise plans, but also you can, more importantly, become convinced that you can do it.

IF IT WERE EASY, EVERYONE WOULD DO IT

The reason why we seldom embrace changes in our diets such as going back to nature and eating foods in their more natural state is because it is unpleasant to think of sacrifice. We just assume it is going to be grueling. Yet no one who attends a Birchcreek retreat, who fully participates in the Birchcreek Jump-Start Your Life program, is disappointed in the food or its preparation. Invariably, after only a few days, people comment on how satisfied they are. People are ecstatic over the myriad of food choices, textures, aromas, and tastes of well-prepared delicious entrées. Nature supplies the "raw materials," and our ingenious human brains, the same ones that got us into trouble, get us out of trouble. Healthy ethnic dishes explode with taste and texture. And people who prefer a blander diet appreciate the subtleties only natural foods can deliver.

Beginning to lose weight for good and to get healthy requires us to address our nutritional deficiencies with logic, common sense, and positive anticipation. This resource will help. It is about time we eat with a little adventure rather than only with salt, sugar, and animal fat. Changing our frame of reference when it comes to food may not be easy, but it is the only way to explore and enjoy nature's bounty. At Birchcreek we have done all the fieldwork and homework. All you have to do is read and learn.

In the years that we've been doing the Birchcreek Jump-Start Your Life program, a couple of things have remained true. For one, we have never had to change the name. Jump-Start Your Life is appropriate. It is a launching point from which you can start again. This program is self-motivating. People stop smoking all the time when they are really motivated. Fewer ice cream or chocolate lovers can just one day decide, "That's it, no more, ever." The people who know what they need to do to lose weight or get healthy might be able to inch their way closer to a more perfect diet, but often it takes a sudden sickness or the threat of a close brush with serious illness to prompt them to treat diet change with urgency and resolve. Even then, when the passion of the moment passes, they often revert to a compromise and eventually recklessly abandon the goal. The Jump-Start Your Life program changes your whole lifestyle. That's why it can bring permanent change.

Your original reason for change may be for vanity, health, or just feeling more comfortable in your own skin. Perhaps you awakened one morning and looked in the mirror and realized how far short you have fallen from what you expected for this time in your life. Once and for all you draw a line in the sand, and you resolve to take no prisoners. You are the kind of person who succeeds! There are no shortcuts. True change starts with a strong decision, and it works itself one step at a time, one day at a time.

The Birchcreek Jump-Start Your Life program has been refined over the years. Our methods of showing people how they can alter their eating lifestyle have become less willpower driven as we have been more able to explain how our bodies work best, so that we can cooperate with the process by providing ourselves with good nutrition. We have added to the program while very seldom subtracting from it. Birchcreek, unlike many other programs, focuses on the biological truths about your physiology. By using human physiology to your advantage, you engage in a mind/body learning experience.

Nothing else is more powerful than equipping you for your own success. This is not a temporary fad diet through which you may reach a temporary goal. Our program helps prevent future failure from the same junk food or other unhealthy patterns that got you in trouble before. We teach you a lifestyle of eating for the rest of your life.

Truthfully there is no way to make the process of changing your eating habits altogether attractive ahead of time. At Birchcreek we will offer you the 100 percent truth regarding diet, lifestyle, and the human condition. It is up to you to adopt as little or as much as you feel you can. You will learn what you should be eating and why and what the ramifications are when you do not. We give our clients a significant advantage over the rest of the population, who lack this vital knowledge and understanding concerning diet and nutrition.

AS WILLIAM WALLACE SAID IN *BRAVEHEART*, "I'VE COME TO PICK A FIGHT!"

Your body is designed to run on certain fuel, and no matter how much you like the taste or you would like to think it is good for you, the food you eat falls into two categories: food that is natural to our species and food that is unnatural. In this case unnatural almost always means bad.

Even as we have made food more attractive or tasty—and less natural—it has become more harmful. Just watch the food commercials on evening television. The focus is taste and price, not nutrition and health. With reckless abandon consumers demand fast and prepackaged food in greater quantities. An industry has taken over our food production, while engineering our tastes to drive us wild. Naturally we want to eat only food that passes our taste test, and in general, Americans tend to avoid foods that might require the acquisition of a particular new taste. We follow sweet and salt blindly as sheep follow each other off a cliff. And to our death we go by the millions per year unnecessarily.

America needs to hear the truth about food. At Birchcreek our philosophy is based in biological truth concerning health and dietary requirements. We are not concerned about how many rooms we fill at any of our resort locations. We tell people that we are going to tell them the truth about what they need to eat in order to be healthy, to lose weight, to regain their vitality, and to live a long and healthy life far into old age. How much benefit they receive will reflect how much or how little of our program they adopt, and our success is driven by their success. We tell them that instead of confusing them with compromises, we want to show them the truth and help them make a plan for how to negotiate this new dietary lifestyle within their capacity to perform it. We say, "So let's assume you are finished with messing around with fad diets. You're finally ready to eat as if it matters, as if your life depends on it. It does."

People are not perfect. It can be difficult to force someone to eat a perfect diet if they have been eating garbage all their lives. Yet when a person comes to understand some basic concepts that never change and cannot be compromised, it can make it easier to adopt some and tweak others.

Each and every person in America is busy, working hard to put food on the table and to pursue their corporate lives and all the variations of career paths. But no one should be too busy to learn new facts about the food on the table. We have never encountered a person whose life situation prevented us from being able to help them develop a way of eating that could fit into their lifestyle.

The Birchcreek Jump-Start Your Life program incorporates recipes for life. These recipes come in the form of food plans, strategies, and adaptable lifestyle changes anyone can implement, one step at a time. As we present them within the pages of this book, you will receive a brand-new knowledge about the nutrition required by your body, and you will come to understand the consequences of the poor choices you have been making for yourself.

ABOUT FACE!

While all of this information may seem to represent the long way out of the maze, it is the only sure way out of the maze. There are no magic bullets. There are no shortcuts. There will not be any scientific inventions in the future that are going to solve the problem of the poor health and obesity in America. The absolute solution is found only in returning to eating the foods that were meant for our bodies, foods that remain in their natural forms and that therefore retain all the elements high in nutrition, such as natural antioxidants, vitamins and minerals, bioflavonoids, and essential fatty acids.

We need to start applying our common sense. As I stated previously, we must note that the animal kingdom is relatively healthy and that wholesale disease and sickness seems to occur uniquely within the human race. Why, out of all the life on this planet, is humankind plagued with such a myriad of diseases and degenerative ailments while the rest of the wild animal kingdom remains relatively free from these diseases?

The answer may lie in the unique ways we choose to prepare our food. For millennia people have been using their intellects to alter their food; this is quite different from the kind of instinctive eating that happens in the animal kingdom. In fact, only humans can permanently and profoundly alter their environment. Forced by necessity and opportunity as well as taste enhancement, only humans take food and alter it with heat, chemicals, and additives, creating for themselves enhanced tastes that are not natural to food.

Although we human beings are special and unique on this planet, we must understand that the basic rules of biology have not been suspended for our category of living beings.

The biological requirements for health and vitality remain the same as they always were, and food products that have been reengineered for convenience or taste often cannot fulfill them.

Just look at how liberally the cooks in every restaurant use sugar and salt. Without using those two key ingredients and combining them with other exotic ingredients to make unique tastes, that restaurant would lose business in a hurry. It is all well and good for you to leave that restaurant with a satisfied palate, but if your biological systems could talk, they would accuse you of crimes against your own humanity.

At Birchcreek we tell people from the very beginning that the problem with our diet is that we have made a hobby out of eating. Hobbies are satisfying. They take up time, and they temporarily settle us. We choose hobbies because we are looking for a release or some kind of pleasure, or for the comfort of having one realm of complete control. As we are seeking a release from the pressures of life, our food not only becomes our habit of choice, fulfilling cravings and compulsions, but also soon it begins to drive every emotion attached to our lives. We eat nervously, for the purpose of fulfilling something that is not being fulfilled and because that eating offers us satisfaction at the most personal and accessible level.

OUR SECURITY BLANKET

Not only have we developed a love affair with food, but we've also developed a love affair with creating a niche in time to enjoy that food. It has become an escape from life. Food has become a safe haven, a satisfaction. When it becomes embedded in the temperament and the constitution of a person, it can become dangerous pattern, very similar to recreational drug use. We live in a society that is littered with disorders, and at the top of the list are the all-too-common eating disorders, which are the product of frustrated physiology. For all of our desire to be the masters of our own universe, when all is said and done, we are controlled by our food.

This being the case, we need to learn how to shift our attention from one type of eating to another—without sacrificing the security that we have derived from our food. This shift can be exciting and rewarding. Birchcreek workshops show how much fun food preparation can be, how easy it can be, and how little time it needs to take. We tackle some of the biggest myths about healthful, natural eating, namely that:

1. It costs more.

2. It takes too much time to prepare.

3. It means sacrificing taste.

In our series of cooking workshops we demonstrate how to put a delicious, natural meal together in about fifteen or twenty minutes whether you are feeding two people or five people. People are amazed when they think they are going to spend forty-five minutes in a workshop and then, even with all the explanation, we are out of there in twenty minutes—and they have even been able to taste all the food that was prepared, both cooked and uncooked. It would be anticlimactic if it weren't so delicious. Eating this way results in eating less and feeling satiated longer. Eating less, and less often, equals reduced costs.

You cannot afford to compromise when considering your health. At Birchcreek we know that if a program works correctly and is offered in a caring, nurturing environment, the results will speak for themselves. That is what has happened, and that is what will continue to happen, with excellence.

PEOPLE JUST LIKE YOU

At Birchcreek we have people from every walk of life. We have had our share of doctors and nurses. You might ask why professional medical people would choose a nonclinical venue such as Birchcreek to shed pounds. After all, they know how to lose weight according to their own knowledge. But they can't seem to do it. They need an environment where they can retreat from their daily lives to accomplish what they know they cannot do on their own. They may be clinically oriented, but they don't need a clinical approach. So they come to Birchcreek specifically for a nonclinical approach to losing a few pounds. When they find our website (www.weightloss retreat.com), it convinces them that this will be a good way to starve a few pounds off in a quiet, out-of-the way place without distractions.

Soon they become well aware that they have gotten more than they originally bargained for. Seminars and workshops address the finer points of the nutritional, scientific, and practical psychology of diet and lifestyle. Clients attend informative, interactive food workshops. After the first day they realize that they might learn something as well as lose something. After one week, when they have witnessed their own bodies' ability to restore health and vitality through detoxification and proper nutrition, they become very enthusiastic. Their results? Renewed energy and rapid weight loss. As our guests they have attended our seminars and listened to this ex-aerospace worker as he begins to unlock the mysteries and the maze of misinformation that they have never understood before. (Some of them, of course, are not concerned with misinformation. They just say, "Get it done.")

In short, Birchcreek is a relaxing retreat focused on health, weight loss, exercise, and rest. Averaging a dozen clients at a time, it is a small and intimate place. Many, perhaps half of the clients, are people who have been to Birchcreek before and who have returned for more. That says a lot.

DON'T REINVENT THE WHEEL

We really have not invented anything. Both Julie and I have been blessed with a logical, engineering approach to life, and we have applied it to the complex principles of physiology and nutrition.

When medical professionals take part in our program, they tell us how refreshing it is to hear a simplified presentation of so much information. We use the commonsense knowledge and understanding of our own human biology to build a model that anyone can follow and comprehend.

When doctors experience the seminars and workshops, with their visual and hands-on applications, they express amazement that they never heard these truths put in the same order that we have. And for the first time in their lives they can implement them. They go away saying, "I'm in the field of medicine, but now I have the ability to express to my patients the reasons why diet is so vitally important for health and restoration." Now doctors can communicate with their patients in normal language instead of in highly synthesized technical terms from science and medicine.

Sometimes doctors refer their patients here because of the reports of their other patients who came independently to Birchcreek and returned with astounding results. The Birchcreek Jump-Start Your Life program places a tremendous emphasis on your body's ability to heal and restore itself. It is designed to put health on the fast track. When you give your body what it needs, especially in the form of the fuel it needs to perform its normal activities, your body will almost always exceed your expectations.

Let's allow our bodies to do what they were designed to do through the food we eat and the lifestyle we live!

CHAPTER 3

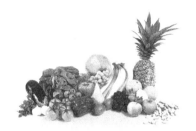

I FEEL SO LOUSY

I am a living testimony of how changing diet and lifestyle can improve overall health. I am about ten years older than my wife. One day Julie looked me straight in the eyes and said, "You know, you look horrible. I can tell that your vitality is gone. You look drained, and you are walking around with aches and pains. When we're in our seventies or eighties, I don't want to have to lift you from the couch to the chair to the bed."

After she said that, I told her, "I should be so fortunate to live that long considering that my father died at sixty-seven and my mom lived the last twelve years of her life fighting cancer and various digestive disorders."

She replied, "I want you to go get a checkup."

When I went to my doctor for a complete physical, I found out that my blood pressure was through the roof, my cholesterol was dangerously high, and my triglycerides were off the chart. I was forty pounds heavier than I am now. I looked as terrible as I felt.

My doctor said that was typical for an American about my age. I was no better and no worse than my peers. I was the average fifty-year-old.

Unfortunately, average isn't normal.

DON'T CROSS-POLLINATE WORDS

We have cross-pollinated the word *average* with the word *normal*. The statistical averages of illnesses in America should not be considered normal. Normal people (who eat properly) do not usually get heart disease, cancers, and diabetes in the numbers that we see in our society. Normal people don't get joint pain, reflux, high blood pressure, and high cholesterol. These are abnormal conditions, and people won't get them unless they work very hard to earn them through a lifestyle of unhealthy eating.

When I went to my doctor, I heard what everyone hears: "We have to get you on medication, and you might have to alter your diet a little bit." I left with a real scare!

However, I knew a man who had been 125 pounds overweight and who had had reflux disease most of his adult life. He had also had precancerous lesions on his esophagus, and he was a type 2 diabetic. In the space of a year he had completely reversed his health and appearance.

He now has a rock-hard body, and he is the picture of health and vitality that most people would attribute to genetics. His name is Steve Wyckoff, and I want to give him the credit he deserves. Not only was he an early convert to a plant-based diet when it was far less popular, but he was also perhaps my greatest motivation to improve my health. I always felt that if I could know someone who did something extraordinary, then I might be able to do it as well. I found out that the extraordinary was not so extraordinary at all, but more real and more ordinary, more natural after all.

When I found my health failing, I got in touch with Steve and said, "I want to do whatever you did to go from where you were to where you are." I had read the statistics and was not impressed with the outlook of controlling my body's functions with medications. I conscripted him to launch me in the direction of whatever he had done to turn his health around.

Within three months I had lost thirty-six pounds. People said that I didn't even look like the same person. I was as surprised at the speed of my transformation as they were. Immediately I invested myself in the study of nutrition and health. I just overwhelmed myself with information about a healthy natural diet and moderate activity, learning about a new lifestyle, and it transformed my life. My doctor even asked me if she could take a look at the materials with which I was so consumed. I gave her the entire package of information that I had accumulated over a six-month period.

Now she has been our doctor on call for our clients over the years, and we have benefited as well from her expertise. On many occasions she has referred her patients to Birchcreek for alternative ways of improving their health.

THE SEESAW OF WEIGHT LOSS

The by-product of healthy eating is rapid, healthy weight loss. The by-product of healthy eating is natural detoxification. It is those two things that can transform your life. If one agrees that health and longevity are largely determined by the food we eat and activity we engage in, then one can conclude that the deficiencies and toxicities in the food we eat and the sedentary lifestyle we live will lead to both premature degenerative diseases and death. Regardless of whether you adopt a different eating and activity lifestyle for rapid, healthy weight loss or for health restoration, our program works every time.

I was watching a TV program about health secrets and what can be done to fix our poor state of health. Five different alternatives to weight loss were presented. Each one of them had a piece of the truth. One person was talking about calories and saying every calorie unburned is a calorie stored as fat. Another was talking about how hormones and the production and stimulation of those hormones through certain foods we eat will in turn stimulate metabolic reactions that will destroy fat. Both were, in part, correct. Another was talking about measuring carbohydrates intake, while still another was talking about getting proper protein and restricting carbohydrates. Well, they are all right to a certain extent too. You see, there are many ways of losing pounds, but there is only one way of getting healthy and reaching your healthy, perfect weight quickly and safely.

The by-products of a healthy lifestyle are: rapid, healthy weight loss; revitalization; rejuvenation; and stimulation of our necessary bodily functions.

The big problem for Americans is that they don't know what

food is healthy. I could ask everyone to list all the foods they eat in the morning, the afternoon, and the evening and put a little heart next to those foods that they perceive to be healthy and an "x" next to those that they perceive to be unhealthy. It would prove to be a difficult assignment, because we really cannot define "healthy food." We are intoxicated by commercials, and we believe branding on products that belies the truth. We read statements that this is "healthy" and that one is "fortified" and this other one is "natural." None of that really means much when you understand the nature of nutrition and what processing does to the vitality and power in foods.

ME AND MY HARLEY

Here's what I have discovered: High Octane = More Mileage, Less Waste.

Any processing of food depletes its power (the "octane"). We really have to concentrate on food that I call high in octane, because high-octane food produces less waste, more power, and better "gas mileage." Who doesn't know that?

I had always wanted a Harley. So when I turned sixty, I bought my first Harley-Davidson. I could not have expected to ride it or to learn how to ride it or feel confident on it if I had still been severely overweight and had never ridden before. But, at sixty years of age, I was in great shape and felt great. I felt young, and I felt there was no reason why I should not be on that bike. I bought it. Very early on I learned that I had to put high-octane fuel in that machine. The manufacturer's recommendation is to use high-test only and never, ever use low-octane fuel. One day I had to take a ride, and I knew that the distance from where I was to where I was going would take a certain number of gallons. Having only a few bucks in my pocket, I decided to put low octane/regular fuel in the bike. Did I ever learn a lesson! It started making noises and stuttering and puttering, and I thought there was something wrong with the engine. So when I got back to town I took it to my dealer, and he looked it over. Everything checked out— except that the plugs were fouled and dirty.

I said, "I don't know what happened. I did what everybody else does; I put gas in it, and I rode." He asked me what kind of gas I used, and I replied that I had put some regular in but I didn't think it would matter much. He then told me that if I used nothing but high-octane fuel in this machine and serviced it according to factory specs, it would last a good long time with little or no trouble. But he warned me that if I put regular gas in it, I would shorten the life of the motor by about 50 percent.

I think of that story now when people come and ask me about the significance of certain food choices in their lives. I tell them it is all about octane. If you think you can feed your body low-octane fuel when it was designed for high-test fuel and not suffer premature problems, you are mistaken.

GARBAGE IN, GARBAGE OUT . . . SOMETIMES

Waste in our bodies, just like waste in any machine, must be removed quickly and efficiently. Any factory creates waste in the process of manufacturing, and a waste removal system must be in place. Our bodies have sanitation departments that eliminate waste and toxic buildup in our bodies. Yet the very organs that take care of the waste produced by the metabolism of the food we eat are directly affected by poor-quality fuel.

You see, even the disposal mechanisms require the correct fuel to operate efficiently. More waste is accumulated when the food we eat is low in octane. In addition, the machinery, the organs involved in elimination, will become overburdened and overwhelmed. Our bodies were not designed to be in continual emergency mode, trying to get rid of waste overload all of the time. Our bodies were not designed to process and eliminate the kinds and volume of waste produced from low-octane foods.

Certain organs of your body—your skin, kidneys, colon, lungs, and mucous membranes—are involved in the process of elimination. They are designed the same way that manufacturers design their waste elimination systems. God, our designer and manufacturer, designed our bodies to get rid of the kinds of waste occurring in the food or the fuel that He has recommended for our bodies. I don't want to keep on deviating from His plan, do you?

CHAPTER 4

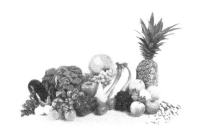

A VERY SAD DIET

For thousands of years the incidence of disease and maladies in the human population has remained infinitely higher than any other species on earth. But in the past 150 to 200 years we have drastically changed our lifestyle of eating. Two hundred years ago the whole world was an agrarian culture. People's lives were knitted to agriculture. But with the spawning of industrialization, things began to change. Still, even my grandmother and her mother and father ate more raw foods than we do today. Of course they cooked much of their food, but they also ate a tremendous amount of raw food: fruits and vegetables, nuts and seeds. Since then we have begun to rely more and more on cooked food and more heavily on meat and dairy. In more recent times we have bought into the message of food commercials and societal norms. Now we're finding out that we have been deceived, and scientific findings are backing that up.

THE BIG MACHINE MEETS LOBBYISTS

Between the scientific community and the general population we have something called government. Scientists are constantly finding out more about the human body, and the legislative branch of the American government is constantly instituting new rules and regulations.

For example, read the side panel on a pack of cigarettes. One of the warning labels states: "Smoking causes lung cancer, heart disease, emphysema, and may complicate pregnancy."[1] The reason that is printed on a pack of cigarettes is that lobbyists, armed with statistics from medical scientists, forced industry lobbyists to withdraw their efforts on behalf of the tobacco industry. Forty-five years ago legislation was passed, and warnings began to be printed on every pack of cigarettes that was manufactured for sale in this country. Today none of us doubt that cigarette smoking and lung cancer are linked. And—let me throw a bomb at you—those same institutions that have identified the link between cigarette smoking and lung cancer are the ones that now say they have found a link between the food we eat and the diseases and premature and chronic conditions from which we suffer. We are not talking about obscure institutions in the corner of our country or in a foreign third world country. We are talking about the same institutions of research that pressured the government to print cancer warnings on each pack of cigarettes.

In fact, there have been sixteen hundred more studies that

have connected the consumption of meat and dairy to heart disease, cancers, diabetes, and osteoporosis than have connected lung cancer to cigarette smoking.[2] We are not talking about the overconsumption of meat and dairy, merely the consumption of them. This is a shock to most people, but that's because, by the time the scientific results reach the public, we hear only a part of the findings.

Let me give you an example of what happens when researchers and lobbyists meet and battle it out. Let's say I have a factory that makes redwood toothpicks. I take one redwood tree and push that redwood tree through a machine; out the other side come the toothpicks. Well, the lobby groups, representing business and government, force me to install a limiting function in the machinery so that when a redwood tree trunk enters on one side, only one toothpick pops out the other side. To judge by the quality of that toothpick, you would declare that the machine is doing what it is supposed to do. But if you would compare the size of the redwood tree to what the machine actually produced, you can see that something is wrong with this picture.

This is a picture of what happens to scientific information as it is pushed through Congress and governmental agencies when company and industry lobbyists do face-to-face battle. They negotiate the truth right out of the product as they begin to protect product profits or product reputation. The existence of the whole "redwood" never gets revealed.

GENETICS IN THE BLEACHERS

Before it reaches us, the information has been sanitized for our consumption. Scientific investigators have found that, although genetics plays a role in the propensity to acquire health problems, the tipping point is toxicity and deficiency caused by a lifetime of eating foods we are not designed to consume. Instead of eating high-octane foods, fruits, and vegetables, we have been relying on low-octane meat, dairy, and cooked foods, as well as chemically processed foods.

As this information has passed through the governmental filters, what we hear on the other end is simply the single toothpick of information: "Eat more fruits and vegetables, and eat less meat and dairy." This pasteurized, neutralized, watered-down, simplistic version of the truth cannot help to improve our health. The average person doesn't really know what to do with that slogan. People don't tend to consume less of the bad stuff and more of the good stuff. Instead they hardly give up any of the bad stuff and merely try to add some of the good stuff. "Maybe I should eat a salad or an apple a day," they say. Well, that's not enough. Our digestive system has been designed to do wonderful things, but we don't feel any different when it is working too hard, do we? We only find out it is working too hard when things begin to break.

IDIOT LIGHTS ON OUR DASHBOARD

Cars today contain a little computer chip. That computer chip governs the operation of that car. It handles the regulation of the gas and air mixture, the RPMs, the coolant system, and even the electrical distribution to the spark plugs. Sometimes it can even order up more or less tire pressure and react to blind spots. Just take a look when you turn the key to the "on" position. See how many lights light up on your dashboard. And when you start your car, all those lights turn off...you hope!

You know that if you were to take your car right as it comes out of a factory and run it according to factory specs and not abuse it, that car would have a long life span. Let's assume you took that car and you drove down into the depths of Death Valley, and then, if it were possible (for the purpose of explanation), you instantly drove it up to the heights of Pikes Peak. Behind the scenes that little computer chip would be regulating the needed gas flow, airflow, RPMs, coolant temperatures, and the electrical spark. Alterations would be taking place, but you wouldn't know they were happening while the car continued to operate perfectly. If you really abuse that car and do crazy things with it and drive it beyond the manufacturer's specifications, idiot lights would begin to warn you that something is not right with that car and that, if you are smart, you should stop and get it checked out. Every one of those lights warns you about some aspect of your car. If the car is not able to regulate normal operation, one of those idiot lights comes on to inform you of a particular problem. No one wants idiot lights to go on. Sometimes they do at the most inopportune times.

I think that human beings come equipped with idiot lights too. Our bodies don't have buttons, gauges, flashing lights, and sirens, but they really do have idiot lights or warning indicators. When your joints ache, an idiot light is going off. When you have gained weight, the scale is an idiot light. When you have acid reflux or your blood pressure or your cholesterol is a little too high or your heart rate is irregular for no apparent reason, those are indicators that something is not working right. When you have headaches or the beginnings of a skin disorder or allergies, it is time for a checkup.

Think of the many kinds of maladies that we are suffering from today that people hardly heard of one hundred years ago, such as fibromyalgia, carpal tunnel syndrome, migraines, Crohn's disease, irritable bowel syndrome, lactose intolerance, exotic allergies, and a host of neurological disorders. These are the idiot lights warning us to stop, or we will severely damage our machine! By the time the diagnosis is made of heart disease or cancer, things are seriously broken.

How do we avoid this? People whose idiot lights are broadcasting warnings can do something about it; they can reverse the cycle—but not by treating the symptoms with medication (and American culture loves its medicine). We love to prescribe pharmaceutical remedies for what ails us. And what do these remedies do? They can relieve discomfort, soothe a pain or inflammation, prevent or reverse infection, and at best deliver to your body an opportunity for your body to heal itself. How is it that the medicine that gets the credit for healing?

We heal from within

You see, we don't heal a broken bone with a cast on our arm. We heal from within. Built into our biology is the ability to heal and restore health, if we give our bodies the opportunity to do what they were well designed to do. That opportunity, however, can never be at an optimum level as long as we are fueling ourselves with the very foods that created the problem. Meantime, the medical field is desperately trying to keep up with the enormous and growing incidence of sickness and disease in this country, and it is questionable whether medicine is winning the battle. One study has stated that children in America today might be the first generation of Americans who will have a shorter life span than their parents.[3]

A DUAL CORE PROCESSOR

The autonomic system of your body knows how to cause the body to heal itself. Your body operates on two levels; it has a somatic system and an autonomic system. Your body relies on the autonomic system to heal, correct, fix, and repair problems. Its functioning is invisible to you, and it happens automatically. The somatic system, on the other hand, is driven by your own volition. You move your limbs, take a drink of water, scribble on a piece of paper, walk, skip, scratch an eye, or brush your hair. You decide to do these things.

You don't have to think about the autonomic system. You are not turning any dials or pressing any buttons to regulate your heart rate, your respiration, your core temperature, the production and distribution of hormones, and cell division in your body. It is like the computer chip in your car. Your autonomic system handles more than 99 percent of the operation of your physical body. Remember the importance of your body's autonomic system, because it is a cornerstone of understanding how your body works, and I will continue to emphasize its importance.

It is this autonomic system that preserves and restores health. If you got lost in a snowstorm and began to suffer from the effects of zero degree temperatures (hypothermia), all the blood in your body would begin to migrate to your internal organs—to preserve your life. Your autonomic system could care less if you lose the tip of your nose, your toes, your earlobes, or your fingertips to frostbite. Your body can lose incidental appendages in the process of preserving your heartbeat, brain function, lung function, and more. Even if your arms and your legs have to be amputated, your autonomic system would have succeeded in helping you to survive that incident.

In much the same way, when you persist in eating the wrong foods, you create so much waste that your body can't remove it. Your body begins to compensate by implementing counter-measures, but these interventions put a strain on your body. Your body was not designed to deal with emergencies for an extended period of time. When it does, the idiot lights begin to flash, and it is time (hopefully not too late) for you to use your volition to make some significant changes in the way you have been treating yourself.

CHAPTER 5

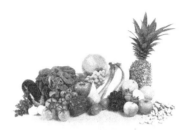

ADJUSTING YOUR FRAME
OF REFERENCE

Today an egg is good for you; last year an egg was bad for you. Today butter is bad, but tomorrow butter may be good. Does the news about food confuse you? Many times marketing drives it. Let's see what scientists have to say about all of this.

Your body runs best on certain foods, and it really doesn't give a hill of beans what you think. It doesn't matter what you wish would happen; if a substance fails to benefit the human body, it is harmful. My mother and grandmother did their best to feed their children, but that doesn't mean they were always right.

BACK TO THE BEGINNING

In order to understand what is really right and wrong for your physiology you need to go back to the point where humans started to eat meat and dairy, which was thousands of years ago, after Adam and Eve were banished from the Garden of Eden.

Thank God for forest fires. Imagine an early man finding a well-burned animal carcass. It smelled different and was manageable. Instead of having to run down game and consume it raw, the man could tear it with his hands and chew it with his teeth. He liked the taste. In the future man would domesticate milk-giving mammals as well. So from very early on, humans were meat and dairy consumers.

Yet we were not well designed for either one. Look at the rest of nature. Human beings are the only creatures that, after being weaned off mother's milk, return to drinking milk, usually the milk of a beast of burden that is born at approximately eighty pounds and grows almost to two thousand pounds in a couple of years. The amount of nutrition in cows' milk qualifies it as a superfood, loaded with essential fatty acids, protein, minerals, calcium, and other nutrients. Is it any wonder that *Homo sapiens* benefit from cows' milk? But maybe that milk is not as good for us as has been advertised. Not in the twenty-first century.

In order to understand this better, let's look at the human digestive system and compare it to that of other animals. Get ready for a true paradigm shift. This new model of understanding will serve to adjust your frame of reference. I will plot a course through this information slowly and carefully.

We need to talk about three categories: carnivores, (meat

eaters), herbivores (plant eaters), and omnivores (eaters of both meat and plants). A few animals are omnivores, and most people believe that that is what human beings are. Be assured that just because you can eat, swallow, digest, and expel waste from both the plant world and the animal world, it does not mean you are a true omnivore. A lion or tiger can, if necessary, live off grain, although he is best suited for meat. However, that does not mean he is an omnivore. Starvation will occur, even in the middle of a cornfield, if he runs out of prey. He simply doesn't have the ability to improvise long term.

A bear is a true omnivore. A bear utilizes a fairly narrow spectrum of plant foods, insects, and larvae during the warm months. When the cold weather begins to approach, bears instinctively begin to put on weight by broadening their spectrum of food choices. Eating fish and other animals helps bears gain the weight needed to sustain them through the long winter hibernation. After living on stored fat, they bulk up again in the spring and then level off their consumption with a lighter diet.

A carnivore is an instinctive meat eater. A lion or a tiger will go hungry without sufficient prey, and they do not have the same intellectual ability as humans to consider alternatives. Human beings eat a widely diversified diet because we can. The capacity of our brains enables us to leave instincts behind and improvise, using our intellects to come up with strategies and tools for obtaining and preparing almost any kind of food item.

Herbivores eat plants. They do not eat meat for two reasons: they are not equipped to chew and digest raw meat, and its taste is unpleasant to them. They would starve if their preferred grass or plant ran out, even if a fresh carcass was right in front of them.

Let's create a table for the details.

CARNIVORES	HERBIVORES	HUMANS
Large pointed teeth for penetrating, puncturing, tearing, and holding prey	Flat molars for the purpose of grinding food	Flat molars for the purpose of grinding food
Large sharp claws for climbing, traction, holding, and tearing prey	Feet designed for walking and standing	More articulated hands and feet than those of herbivores, but unable to claw through a carcass
"Sweat" through the tongue, pant to cool off; e.g., dogs	Sweat through their skin; e.g., horses	Sweat through their skin
Acidic saliva, well suited for breaking down flesh	Alkaline saliva, well suited for breaking down nuts, seeds, berries, fruits, and vegetables	Alkaline saliva
Protein enzyme in mouth to help break down flesh	Carbohydrate enzyme in mouth to help break down nuts, seeds, berries, fruits, and vegetables	Carbohydrate enzyme in mouth
Stomach acid high in hydrochloric acid (Hcl)	Stomach acid twenty times less acidic than stomach acid of carnivore	Stomach acid twenty times less acidic than stomach acid of carnivore

You can begin to understand from a biological viewpoint how the attributes of each type determine the best-suited foods.

There are other significant differences between carnivores and herbivores. Look at the digestive tract of the typical carnivore. It has a mouth, an esophagus, a stomach, a relatively short and direct intestinal tract, and an "exhaust pipe." An herbivore also has a mouth, an esophagus, a stomach, and an "exhaust pipe," but a very long, convoluted and winding intestinal tract. Likewise, a human has a mouth, an esophagus, a stomach, an exhaust pipe, and a very long and convoluted intestinal tract.

The length of the carnivore digestive tract is about three to five times its own body length, which leads us to believe that the food going in exits the body as quickly as possible. The length of the digestive tract of a herbivore is ten, twelve, or more times its body length, which leads us to believe that food entering this digestive tract is designed to remain in that digestive tract as long as possible to get the most out of that food. For the same reason, human beings have a digestive tract that is ten to twelve times their body length.

When carnivores ingest food, the food takes four to eight hours to pass from the mouth to out of the body, with a few exceptions. When a herbivore eats food, it takes between twelve to fifteen hours for that food to pass out of its body. Human beings fall into the same category as herbivores; their food digestion takes twelve to fifteen hours.

A carnivore takes down its prey and begins to devour it, in many cases, while it still has life or soon after its death. It rips open the contents of the stomach and eats the contents of that stomach, laps up the blood, and may begin to devour the organs. It would prefer to take the fleshy remains of that animal and stick them up in a tree or bury them, not only to preserve them from other predators but also for the purpose of decomposition. In the process of decomposition, bacteria proliferate, digesting and creating waste of their own, which is highly acidic.

Both bacteria and acid are aggressive deconstructionists. In the carcass they break down the carbohydrates, fats, and proteins to their amino constituent forms. Carnivores, with their short digestive tracts, need flesh that is in a state of decomposition in order to quickly obtain nutrition in the bloodstream. Carnivores are well equipped to deal with this proliferation of bacteria. Humans, however, are ill equipped and would be overcome with toxic poisoning if they ate like true carnivores. In the mouth and stomach of a carnivore, acid helps begin the breakdown and metabolizing of flesh. The protein enzyme in the mouth of carnivores also helps begin to process, metabolizing the nutrition in the meat as it begins to disassemble the protein. The nutrition passes from the intestinal tract to the bloodstream, and the animal's immune system has been perfected so that it does not revolt against the process.

Herbivores, on the other hand, chew their food in order to keep it in the digestive system as long as possible, drawing from the food the maximum amount of nutrition by pulling it through the cellular membrane of the digestive tract and passing it into the bloodstream. What is left over is fiber and waste.

The digestive process of a human being works in much the same way. Because it takes twelve to fifteen hours for food to pass through the digestive tract, the food gets thoroughly depleted of its nutrition. In addition, bacteria do not exist in plant food to the degree it does in rotting flesh.

CONNECT THE DOTS

Let's use our common sense. The leading causes of our sickness, disease, obesity, and dysfunction are deficiency and toxicity derived from a diet that we are not designed for yet we insist on eating.

We want to be told what is good and what is bad, but we need to have more understanding. Most of us are not scientists who are able to read the dry, sophisticated language of study after study. As we try to figure out what the lobbyists are doing and comprehend what really goes on behind the closed doors of the meat and dairy industries, we wonder if any of the other food businesses are on the consumer's side. How can we hear the truth that will set us free?

The reason Birchcreek is so successful is because it has managed to assemble the facts and the evidence in a way that makes perfect sense to the average person. Your most important characteristic is your common sense. Please, don't suspend your common sense because you don't understand the language. If your doctor can't explain your condition and answer all your questions in normal, understandable English, get a new doctor. The medical field has done a dismal job of trying to translate technical, medical jargon into regular language.

We have to put medical terminology in the same category as judicial or contract language. We are not ashamed to ask our lawyers to translate legalese into English, so why do we not ask to have medical conditions and remedies explained and described in whatever detail we need in order to make clear decisions?

I spoke at a nurses' conference recently, and in the audience were a few doctors and researchers. I led two forty-five-minute seminars, one after the other. When I was finished, a doctor said to me, "I wish I could repeat what you've said so my patients would have an easier way of understanding things." He added, "I come from a very technical background that I can't convert into natural, everyday vernacular."

Then a researcher came up and said, "Boy, where have I been?" These professionals know more than I do, but what I had managed to do was to assemble the information so that the average person could understand it.

People will not get insights if they can't understand the facts. The "how and why" and "what to do" answers need to be delivered in intelligible ways. Once a person has formed a clear picture, either through demonstration or words, that person will begin to gain confidence and employ common sense to make decisions. At last change can occur. When this approach gets applied to matters of nutrition, results are rapid and dramatic.

YOUR NEW MODEL OF UNDERSTANDING

It is safe to say that human nature usually dictates our direction. What do I mean by that statement? Whether or not you are aware of the reasons for your decisions, you are motivated by basic survival instincts. Your autonomic system is in control of survival while your somatic system, which includes your free will, helps you make right choices. Each and every day your actions in almost every aspect of life are on trial. When it comes to food, if it tastes good, we repeat that choice. Food must first pass your taste test.

The industrialization of our food supply has eliminated the nutritional value of food. In the twenty-first century food is an energy bar, soft drinks and energy drinks, a box of cereal, fast food, fried food, packaged and powdered foods, snacks, rice cakes, or something to which we add water. Two hundred years ago these might not have been accepted as "food" at all. With a little investigation we might be surprised to learn that these choices are still not considered proper nutrition. Yet much of our population today relies on these convenient foods.

Why, on a standard American diet, are children and adults getting sicker than ever before? If you want to know what the future generation's health is going to be like, weigh your children. It is pretty evident that today's youth are obese. Statistically over 30 percent of American children between the ages of six and nineteen are overweight, with at least half of those being so overweight that they can be classified as obese. In the past twenty-five or thirty years the obesity rate has doubled in young children and tripled in teenagers. As a result the diseases that were once associated only with adults, such as type 2 diabetes, high blood pressure, respiratory and circulatory problems, joint diseases, and even cirrhosis of the liver, are on the rise among children. Needless to say, this obesity epidemic is one of the prime contributors to the nation's soaring health care costs.[1]

In 2006 our nation's estimated spending on obesity-related health care was close to $177 billion. Eighty-three percent of every health care dollar is spent toward the problems that are generated from obesity in both children and adults. Obesity is the primary cause of the nation's top killer, cardiovascular disease.[2] Cardiovascular disease can be almost totally avoided by reducing or eliminating the consumption of meat. We know that harmful cholesterol results from the consumption of meat. What does this say to us?

Another significant problem is lack of exercise. Young people spend too much of their time indoors surfing the web, playing video games, chatting and tweeting and in general engaging with the outside world by electronic means. Physical education has plummeted in popularity and availability. Between 1991 and 2003 enrollment in high school gym classes fell from 42 to 29 percent. It appears that overweight children have at least a 70 percent chance of becoming overweight adults. Fast food can be blamed for much of the problem. The more than 300,000 fast-food restaurants in the United States market inexpensive, high-calorie, high-fat food. A McDonald's Big Mac and a medium order of fries, for example, supplies about a thousand calories. Add to that a large soft drink, loaded with sugar or artificial sweeteners, and you have a killer menu plan—literally.[3]

As I stated in chapter 4, life expectancies are beginning to lose ground to medicine's ability to keep us alive. Studies report that, astonishingly, the present generation's youth are in jeopardy of having a lower life expectancy than their parents.[4] If the trend in childhood obesity continues, experts predict that over the next few decades life expectancy averages will go down by five years.[5] While pharmaceutical companies continue to create new and powerful medicines, we see no commensurate improvement in the prevention and reversal of disorders.

It is evident to me that if our clients who are dependent on blood pressure medications, cholesterol medications, and diabetic medications were deprived of their medicine, their decline would be swift and sure. My personal experience with clients fifty-five years of age and older convinces me that physical problems would cascade rapidly—from potentially dangerous to imminently life threatening—if these clients went without their medications. Medications save lives, but at what cost? A person on prescription medication has to deal with the growing concerns of side effects and dependency on meds rather than solving the root problem.

What should we do? While our problems worsen, we are relying on medicine to make us comfortable. For example, medicines for controlling diabetes leave very little reason for a person to watch what he or she eats. By increasing the medication dosage, a person can then eat anything. A person who takes heart medicine, rather than changing the kinds of foods that create plaque and arterial clogs, can rely on his or her health care provider to medicate as indicated. All these medicines are doing is to help to prevent damage done by dangerously poor diets. They also serve to subvert the auto-nomic system's response to correct or regulate these problems. We are making a very big mistake when we try to trick our very physiology.

THE "WHY" FACTOR

Repeatedly we hear, "Eat more fruits and vegetables! Eat less meat and dairy!"

What are you supposed to do with these statements? You have heard it and have come to believe it, but how do you know how much is required? The word *more* can mean dif-ferent things to different people. If somebody would tell us why, could we understand better how much to change, add, or alter our consumption of fruits and vegetables?

"Eat more!"

"Why?"

If you add an apple a day, have you followed the advice? Is eliminating meat and dairy better than limiting them? We have more questions than answers. It is not about having a wholesome meal once in a while. It is about changing our eating lifestyle so that a poor meal occurs only once in a while. No one is perfect. But the more you learn about your own body, the more you will give your autonomic system the opportunity to repair and restore your body and mind to optimum health.

In their ground-breaking book on diets and disease, authors T. Colin Campbell and Thomas M. Campbell II declare the following:

> After a long career in research and policy making, I now understand why Americans are so confused. As a taxpayer who foots the bill for research and health policy in America, you deserve to know that many of the common notions you have been told about food, health, and disease are wrong.
>
> - Synthetic chemicals in the environment and in your food, as problematic as they may be, are not the main cause of cancer.
>
> - The genes that you inherit from your parents are not the most important factors in determining whether you fall prey to any of the ten leading causes of death.
>
> - The hope that genetic research will eventually lead to drug cures for diseases ignores more powerful solutions that can be employed today.

- Obsessively controlling your intake of any one nutrient, such as carbohydrates, fat, cholesterol, or omega-3 fats, will not result in long-term health.

- Vitamins and nutrient supplements do not give you long-term protection against disease.

- Drugs and surgery don't cure the diseases that kill most Americans.

- Your doctor probably does not know what you need to do to be the healthiest you can be.[6]

Does this help you see why we need to adjust our frame of reference? Our very lives, and the lives of our children, are at stake.

CHAPTER 6

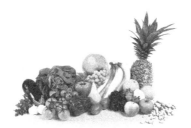

THE LIFE AND POWER
OF LIVING FOODS

he Bible tells a story of a place that was designed just for humans, a place where they could flourish and indulge themselves to their hearts' content. I find it very interesting that in this ancient story a *garden* was the place where God set it up for men and women to derive all their nourishment. (See Genesis 1:29.) As far as we know, the first humans didn't even cook their food; it consisted of the raw fruits of the various trees and plants.

Today when we go back to an all-plant diet, it seems radical, and yet it seems to match the master plan. When we do so, we can expect our entire physiology to change and improve. What happens when you eat a diet based on plant foods? First, the viscosity of your blood changes, because you have started receiving nutrition in a purer, more efficient way than you did when you ate processed foods, cooked foods, and foods that are not well designed for your intestinal tract. Every physical function, every organ, every process your miraculous body undertakes improves vastly. Your body becomes increasingly resistant to sickness and disease.

I have not met one person who has not benefited dramatically from switching from a diet of meat, dairy, and mostly cooked foods to a diet of living, high-octane plants from the cornucopia of food plants that are available to us, both raw and cooked.

And why do we feel so lousy when we indulge in the standard American diet of meat, dairy, and mostly cooked and processed foods? Permit me to describe the primary reason for all that ails us.

STICK WITH LIVING FOOD

We operate best on living food. Living food is food that contains the nutrition in its natural state accompanied by the enzymes that help unlock the nutrition and ready it for absorption and utilization. The enzymes in food are literally the little factories that help disassemble the amino acids of carbohydrates, fats, proteins, and glucose. When a mineral such as calcium, which is produced by nature right out of the ground, is in its natural state, it has an enzyme bonded directly to the molecule.

Carbohydrates, fats, proteins, and natural sugars in raw foods are accompanied by free enzymes that can be borrowed from other foods or that can be manufactured by our own bodies. This will prove to be very significant knowledge to have as we begin to describe the process of digestion and the implications concerning our poor diets.

Living food is food that can and will continue to ripen after it is picked. Ripening is essentially a decomposition process, and this process involves the disassembling of all aspects of nutrition to their smallest constituent forms. This breakdown is what causes a tomato, peach, or banana to continue to ripen when it is picked prematurely.

When you add sugar and acid together, it begins to ferment, yielding alcohol. We know that we can make alcohol out of any living food. You can make banana, cabbage, or barley alcohol. While plants decompose, the combination of sugar and acids promotes a chain reaction and fermentation, with alcohol as the by-product. (Thank goodness our bodies pass fluids in and out, or we would eventually reach a stage of fermentation ourselves. Because we drink and eat and then get rid of our waste, we short-circuit the process of developing alcohol.)

What precedes the alcoholic result is a rise in acidity, which is our mortal enemy. We need to eat foods that produce less acidity, less waste. As it happens, low-octane fuel or foods that do not transfer their energy as efficiently as higher-octane foods create waste that either ferments or is stored by our bodies. The waste by-products increase in their acid content, resulting in an imbalance in the pH of our bodies. Autonomic biology takes care of the problem, but not for long. You see, the poor diets we habitually embrace are like traveling down a one-way street, an express lane to poor health.

The highest-octane food we can put in our bodies is the food that contains the vitamins, minerals, essential fatty acids, bioflavonoids, and complex carbohydrates in the natural form our bodies require for proper operation.

The cooking process diminishes the vitality in our food. It is not that cooked food delivers bad nutrition; it is just inefficient, lower-octane nutrition compared to what it was before it was cooked.

A small amount of heat destroys enzymes, even a few minutes at about 108 degrees. Without these enzymes, the digestion of food is impeded. What are enzymes? They are amino proteins that act like little factories, deconstructing nutritional molecules for use within our bodies. Enzymes are very much like deconstruction crews who break down the nutrition in foods so that we can reorganize and reuse these nutritional aspects as needed. All enzymes are proteins, but all proteins are not enzymes.

Our bodies possess the ability to manufacture and produce these same enzymes. We call them digestive enzymes. Our bodies can make carbohydrate, fat, protein, and glucose enzymes.

Minerals and metals are not included in that list. An inert product such as calcium must be absorbed and metabolized before it is flushed out by our waste management system. When foods containing calcium are consumed in their raw form, the enzyme connected to the mineral molecule does a rapid job of breaking down the calcium. This produces a very important alkaline ash that helps balance our pH; this alkaline ash is really a critical part of our chemistry. In fact, it can be considered a hinge pin of our chemistry—and it is that hinge pin that we have eliminated by destroying its enzyme with heat.

Not only are Americans, on average, calcium deficient, they

are also deficient in high-quality protein, complex carbohydrates, and essential fatty acids. You say to yourself, "How can that be? Look at how much we eat. Something must be wrong with that statement!" The statement happens to be true, and I will be explaining more as we go along.

THE EVER-CHANGING FOOD PYRAMID

The nutritional food pyramid that we grew up with has been drastically revised and can be summarized in the mantra "Eat more fruits and vegetables, and eat less meat and dairy." The new and revised pyramid depicts changes in food positions and quantities that just a decade ago would have seemed incorrect. Of course, our interpretation of that statement, as well as our comprehension of the revised recommendations, could use some updating and revision if it is going to be useful. We need to take a close look at what it means.

About two hundred years ago, living that agrarian lifestyle I mentioned earlier, most people were fit. Their lifestyles were energetic, and they ate better-quality foods than we eat today. Much of the time the food was in an uncooked form.

If you ask people today how much "raw" food they eat, most would say they don't eat any raw food except the occasional piece of fruit or raw salad. They might add that they eat seeds and nuts, but even most of the seeds and nuts they eat are roasted. We have established that we need a certain quality of nutrition in order to live healthy lives. And when we cook everything we eat, we end up diminishing the vitality of that nutrition.

We have also learned that our bodies come equipped to summon our own internally produced digestive enzymes and that active digestive enzymes release the nutrition in food so that our bodies can use it. Without active digestive enzymes you would get the same nutrition out of chewing on Styrofoam! In fact, without enzymes existing in every living animal or vegetable cell, all life on earth would cease to exist.

Enzymes break down the molecules of carbohydrates, fats, proteins, or glucose in order to release the nutrition to our bloodstreams. Enzymes are designed to do their job quickly. Consider the fact that food is constantly moving from the nutrition extraction portion of our digestive systems to the eliminative portion of our digestive systems. Enzymes act quickly to deconstruct nutrition so that we can readily reutilize it for our physiological needs. They serve as the building blocks of continued health by building, restoring, repairing, and nourishing our living bodies.

Cooking, however, destroys these enzymes, which means that our bodies must activate the autonomic process that causes our own enzymes to deconstruct and distribute the nutritional assets in the food we have eaten.

ONCE UPON A TIME

Once upon a time we were introduced to two items that seemed to be both necessary and beneficial to our lives—meat and dairy. As a nation we have been brought up on and are dependent on meat and dairy perhaps more than any other civilization in history. In the later part of the twentieth century it became more and more apparent that this love affair might be harmful to our well-being. It has become increasingly clear that we have come to a significant crossroads in our long relationship with our companions meat and dairy.

Scientists' reports tell us that we were seriously mistaken concerning our food friends. In fact, we find that they may never have been true friends after all, but rather they are squatters who have been taking up just too much room in our dietary lives.

Since we must rely on something, why not rely on our common sense? Let's not reinvent the wheel. Let's get back to obtaining, preparing, and eating our food in the most basic ways possible.

DON'T SUSPEND YOUR COMMON SENSE

If you think about it, you realize that we are the only beings on this planet who cook our food and eat outside of the instinctive package we were created and designed for. Our brain has the ability to improvise. As I have been explaining, we can choose to eat not only the good foods but also foods that are not well suited for our species, with meat and dairy being the biggest culprits. Invariably someone will question me on this, because people have been eating meat and dairy for thousands of years. Why all of a sudden is it bad? It hasn't become bad all of a sudden; it is just that we have finally been able to figure out *why* it is bad, so that we can revert to healthier ways of feeding ourselves.

Historically we see signs of human health in the fossil record. Deficiencies in certain essentials show up in skeletal deformations and in the examination of the teeth and bones of ancient people. It seems that the ability of human beings to diversify and innovate sometimes helped them manage to keep one step ahead of chronic and severe nutritional deprivation, while at other times in history deprivation resulted in wholesale ailments and diseases. People, in their struggle for life, oftentimes found themselves deep inside uncharted nutritional territory.

When humans began to rely on meat and dairy for food, much of their nutritional needs were met. But the introduction of meat and dairy initiated, in a sense, a race against time. This race was between our bodies' inability to easily handle these new foods and our bodies' natural ability to adapt or evolve. In this case our physiology could have used an additional several million years to adapt if we are to adopt an old earth model. Instead we have had thousands of years, which is not enough time to physically adapt to this new and difficult process of digesting meat and dairy.

PASTEURIZATION AND FOOD PROCESSING

In the early 1960s medical statistics began to show that the health of Americans had become significantly worse than in previous decades. Instead of it being a crest of a wave that broke on a couple of bad years, the poor health of America appeared more like a tsunami of illness. An entire generation was entering middle age, sicker than ever before in recorded history. Both the level of disease and degenerative symptoms and the rate of incidents of these disorders were higher than ever before, and people began to try to find out why. Why were heart disease, dangerous cholesterol, diabetes, high blood pressure, cancers, and many other maladies appearing in such large numbers? The scientists of the day began to look at what societal changes may have brought about this development.

They began to hone in on a particular problem caused by industrialization in America, which started in the 1800s and continued well into the 1900s. As local farms gave way to large-scale operations, food distribution became a new concern. When transporting food to faraway locations, how could it be kept safe? Shelf life became the primary challenge. Of course, refrigeration played a large role in retarding the spoilage of foods, but what took place, especially in our dairy industry, that changed the course of nutrition in America?

When I was a young boy, nine or ten years old, I lived outside of Manhattan in a little neighborhood in Queens, New York. A poultry farm and a dairy farm were within a five-minute walk from our home, and I used to walk to them with my grandfather. We were sent out every couple of days to pick up fresh produce, dairy products, and meat. My grandmother had immigrated from Italy when she was twelve years old. Even in Manhattan, where her family lived, she could still obtain much of her food the same way as she had in Italy as a child, where she could walk to the home of a local farmer.

Obviously, now there are no more farms within walking distance of these neighborhoods. Even if farms were within walking distance today, chances are that what they would sell wouldn't resemble what Grandma used to buy. Because of population growth and industrialization, goods now need to be shipped in from outside the city, and in order to last long enough, much of it has had preservatives added. In the case of milk and other dairy products, we now have pasteurization, which kills off any harmful bacteria that may have found their way into the system—as well as those powerful enzymes I have been describing.

Once upon a time milk could be considered a wonder food because of its broad spectrum of nutrition and its power to aid digestion. When combined in the intestines with meat, which can be very difficult for the human system to break down, milk could help facilitate digestion. Active enzymes in unpasteurized milk, along with a healthy amount of naturally forming bacteria, helped digest the fats in dairy and the flesh of meat. The presence of those enzymes also kept people's bodies from needing to use up their own digestive enzymes.

As you know, people have been eating meat and drinking unpasteurized milk for thousands of years. Just think what a sudden dependency on our own enzyme bank accounts was demanded when we started pasteurizing milk and essentially unplugged this naturally potent source of digestive enzymes found in unpasteurized dairy products! In addition, consumption of raw fruits and vegetables started decreasing as modernization and industrialization escalated.

Meat and dairy are similar in the type of nutrition they provide. The carbohydrates, fats, and protein in meat are the same carbohydrates, fats, and proteins resident in milk. Milk can be considered liquid meat in a way, except that it is so much more powerful and with greater density than meat. The problem begins with heat. When we cook our meat, we kill off much of the bacteria and all of the active enzymes, rendering meat very difficult to move through the human digestive system. On the other hand, unpasteurized milk, when ingested with the cooked meat, helps to digest the meat by contributing its active enzymes. Enter more heat—pasteurization. Now both types of food have had their enzymes deactivated.

We need to understand more about the way enzymes work in order to remedy the problem. Our bodies will thank us with new vitality as we learn how to return to a diet that better resembles the one we were created to live on.

CHAPTER 7

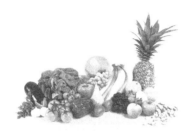

YOUR ENZYME BANK ACCOUNT—THE WEAK LINK

All food, any food, in its natural form contains 100 percent of its nutritional value; none of it is compromised or damaged. The problem is, we almost never eat our food in its natural form. For decades we have been told that the foods we are eating are exceptionally good for us, when in actuality they are only marginally good for us, and some are very bad for us. This misinformation has led many Americans down a destructive path.

In the late 1940s, at the end of World War II, food shelf life became a serious topic of focus. Methods were established to insure the safety of our national food supply although the implications of what was being done to the nutritional value of those foods were not considered. As a result, instead of contributing to the health of Americans, the future health of American citizens was jeopardized.

In the beginning of the Kennedy administration the president was told of the tsunami of health issues that were affecting Americans. The administration needed to get a handle on the source of the problem and find out the impact on the health industries, while at the same time protecting the public. Because obesity in school-age children was on the increase, steps were initiated to combat it. An organization called the President's Council on Physical Fitness was formed, and the council developed a physical fitness test. When that test was given to school-aged children in the early 1960s, approximately 80 percent of all children were able to pass it. However, when that same test was given in the early 2000s, over 80 percent of school-aged children could not pass it.[1]

What happened in those forty years? Why have we continued to see the same health problems, only in an ever-magnified form? Could it have something to do with the actual available nutrition in our food supply?

SNOWBALL EFFECT

How do you build a snowman? You start with a small handful of snow and form a ball and roll it until it becomes so large that you can hardly move it. Obviously the next ball must be smaller because you have to get it up on top of the first one. As you know, if you have ever rolled a snowball downhill, it picks up speed, volume, strength, and force as it gets bigger and bigger.

Like a giant snowball, our national health problem has snowballed and gotten worse. And we can't seem to stop it.

Because of the lack of usable knowledge, the average person does not know how to correct his course. He doesn't know how to make a change. Where food and nutrition are concerned, Joe Average is locked into a lifestyle of taste satisfaction and driven by hunger.

One easily missed fact is that heating food, the act of cooking food, reduces considerably the nutritional value. Cooking diminishes the vitality of the carbohydrates, fats, and proteins. When did this fact slip into the unknown? If you cook a carrot to death, there's far less nutrition in it. The heat and the cooking time reduces the nutritional value by at least 50 percent, as shown below:

50 PERCENT LOSS OF NUTRITIONAL VALUE AFTER COOKING

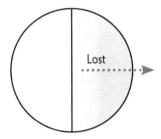

Please understand we still receive some nutrition from cooked foods. And certain foods we have learned to soak and cook, like lentils and legumes, make up an important part of our nutritional requirements. In their case cooking releases and enhances the usable nutrition.

THE LAW OF ADAPTIVE SECRETION OF DIGESTIVE ENZYMES

Now, in addition to recognizing the nutritional value lost to cooking, we must consider in detail the importance of enzymes. In his book *Enzyme Nutrition,* Dr. Edward Howell explains what we know about digestive enzymes.

> In 1943, the physiological laboratory of Northwestern University established the Law of Adaptive Secretion of Digestive Enzymes by experiments on rats. The amount of digestive enzymes secreted by the pancreas in response to carbohydrate, protein, and fat was measured, and it was found that the strength of each enzyme varied with the amount of each of these food materials it was called upon to digest....The Law of Adaptive Secretion of Digestive Enzymes holds that the organism values its enzymes highly and will make no more than are needed for the job. If some of the food is digested by enzymes in the food, the body will make less concentrated digestive enzymes. The Law of Adaptive Secretion of Digestive Enzymes has since been confirmed by dozens of university laboratories throughout the world.[2]

The startling fact is that our enzyme "bank account" is finite, and the faster we use enzymes, the faster they disappear. And there is a consequence to losing them. It has been estimated that if you eat the standard American diet for forty years of your life, which is about half of your projected life expectancy, with very little reliance on raw food, you could deplete as much as half of your digestive enzyme bank account.

The effect is a further 50 percent reduction in your ability to break down and metabolize food. Because enzyme digestion is a time-related process that must be accomplished rather early in the digestive process, the opportunity for complete nutritional release is lost. That means that by the age of forty you will only be capable of deriving 50 percent of the *remaining* nutrition because of your depleted and overworked enzyme bank account, leaving a mere 25 percent of the original nutritional value. As you might expect, deriving only 25 percent nutrition from your food is really going to affect your body. Here's another simple picture of what I'm talking about:

75 PERCENT LOSS OF NUTRITIONAL VALUE FROM EATING COOKED STANDARD DIET FOR FOUR DECADES

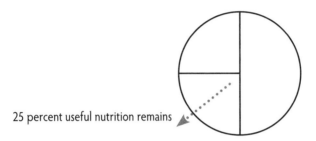

25 percent useful nutrition remains

ONLY SO MUCH IN THE BANK ACCOUNT

Our enzyme banking account has transactions—but they're all withdrawals. We use up some of our lifetime supply of digestive enzymes every time we cook our food, destroying the enzymes in the heating process. This is part of the autonomic system of our bodies, and it is incredibly sensitive and delicate. Your body's autonomic system identifies the viability of enzymes in food as the food passes over receptors in the mouth and on the tongue. It identifies whether or not there are active or deactivated enzymes present. Deactivation means the enzyme has been damaged beyond repair and destroyed by the heating (cooking) process. When this happens, your body will "order up" the production of the proper enzyme.

Carbohydrate enzymes are specific to carbohydrates. They don't help break down fats or proteins. Fat enzymes are specific to fats. They do nothing to help carbohydrates or proteins. Protein enzymes are specific to protein. Glucose enzymes are specific to glucose, and so forth. They do nothing to other aspects of nutrition. The enzymes are married to the family in which they are usable.

In the past we thought these enzymes were produced like blood cells, as needed. They are not! It is as if someone gave you a million dollars when you turned eighteen, with the stipulation that this would be all the money you would receive for the rest of your life. The faster you use it, the faster you lose it. It is not an infinite supply of money.

Our enzyme bank accounts of enzymes are exactly like that—finite. As I stated above, the faster we use our enzymes, the faster we lose them. We never get to redeposit. It is a one-way street, with the average middle-aged American's bank account severely depleted.

The most dangerous aspect of the foods in the typical American diet is the cumulative effect of consuming them for twenty and thirty years. Later in life a person's ability to process these foods diminishes, especially the ability to break down fats. In order to understand the complexity of catabolism of fat in the intestinal tract, we need an explanation of what happens when our body deals with these fats.

Dietary fats consist of complex molecules (lipids) that are not water soluble, and they take longer to digest than carbohydrates or proteins. Fat-digesting enzymes in the mouth and stomach are insufficient for the job, but the pancreas sends more to the duodenum (the upper part of the small intestine) where, with the assistance of bile (produced in the liver and stored in the gallbladder), they emulsify (or divide) the lipid molecules so that the fat-digesting enzymes can divide them into fatty acid and glycerol droplets. Within ten or fifteen minutes nutrition from the fat can be absorbed into the bloodstream through the villi, the large number of tiny "fingers" that cover the inner walls of the small intestine. Once in the bloodstream, the fatty acids migrate to either muscle cells (to be oxidized for energy) or the adipose cells (to be stored as body fat). The human body has been designed to prefer glucose as its source of energy, and only a very small part of the fatty acids get absorbed as glycerols (eventual glucose). As a result a larger proportion of fats will end up being stored as body fat.

A DIGESTIVE EMERGENCY

Our digestive systems, for most of our lives, have been absorbing animal fats. What happens when you impregnate a very porous membrane with animal fat? You're going to reduce its absorption. Picture water being poured through a piece of cheesecloth. That illustrates the condition of a healthy intestinal tract. The water-soluble nutrients pass through the intestinal wall and on into the bloodstream while the rest is evacuated out via the colon. But when animal fats comprise a large proportion of the diet for the first forty years of life, a depreciated enzyme bank account can leave behind insoluble fats and debris within the intestinal membrane, creating a reduction in permeability and absorption. If you were to saturate that cheesecloth with animal fat at a 98.6-degree temperature and then pour water through it, you would probably reduce its permeability by at least 50 percent. In the case of your small intestine, that could mean 50 percent less nutritional absorption.

Our dietary patterns have created a serious digestive emergency. First, the ability of our bodies to begin the breakdown of animal fats earlier on in the digestive cycle has been greatly compromised by the lack of digestive enzymes, and second, animal fats that are not sufficiently broken down are being absorbed into the digestive membranes, rendering the membranes not only less absorbent but also feeding harmful bacteria, which can create even more deleterious ramifications such as "leaky gut syndrome."

FURTHER LOSS OF NUTRITION-ABSORBING CAPACITY

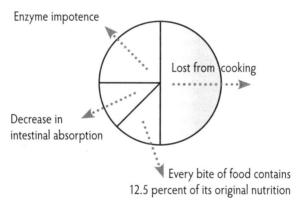

Enzyme impotence

Lost from cooking

Decrease in intestinal absorption

Every bite of food contains 12.5 percent of its original nutrition

This constitutes an emergency situation. A middle-aged person who eats the standard American diet stands to gain only about 12.5 percent of the nutrition from every bite of food he or she takes! No wonder we have such voracious appetites. Our bodies demand more food to make up for the limited nutrition they are getting continually. We start to eat for "fun" even when we are not hungry. Are you beginning to understand?

This is why poor diets and weight gain will forever be

inseparable in an industrialized country such as America. Our bodies require a baseline level of nutrition in order to run the machinery and preserve health. With all of the extenuating circumstances, such as enzyme deficiencies and decreased intestinal absorption, that baseline level can be increasingly difficult to obtain. As we eat more and more, we become more sluggish and less likely to burn off those excess calories. The result: weight gain and ill health. This is where we must change our point of view, our frame of reference, and our model of understanding.

TURNING IT AROUND

All is not lost. The Birchcreek Jump-Start Your Life program can reverse this dangerous condition. I will be describing it in detail in the remainder of this book.

In order to get a jump start on solving the problem, we advise a program of juices derived from fruit and vegetables. The cornerstone of the program is a diet of raw foods, including freshly made juices that not only taste good but also act as natural detoxifiers. They loosen the debris and the fat in your digestive system. They begin to break down the fat that is impregnated in the walls of your intestinal tract and force it into your bloodstream where your immune system can finally take care of it. Because you are not introducing more animal products into your system while you are on the Birchcreek program, your system finally has an opportunity to move the toxins, debris, and animal fat out of your intestinal membranes. Absorption is restored to 100 percent in less than a week! That old cycle of 50 percent depletion in absorption is reversed. No longer are you getting only 12.5 percent total nutrition, but you have regained absorption back up to the 25 percent rate, and that percentage will continue to increase.

RECOVERY OF NUTRITION-ABSORBING CAPACITY

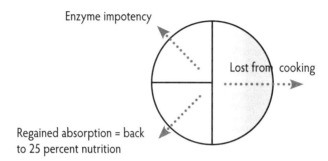

The living (uncooked) food you eat on the Birchcreek program is very rich in enzymes. Now, because you are utilizing the natural enzymes in living food juices, nutrition can be unlocked. You are able to metabolize 100 percent of the enzyme-rich food that you are eating or drinking raw. In addition, you are no longer withdrawing from your depleted enzyme bank account.

Furthermore, because you are no longer cooking your food, you are no longer diminishing its vitality. Every bite or swallow of pure vegetable or fruit juice gives you the full potency of its nutrition. *Soon you will be back at 100 percent!*

RAW FOOD ADVANTAGE =100 PERCENT NUTRITIONAL RELEASE

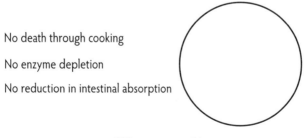

In summary, eating more raw food than cooked food ensures:

1. Enhanced nutritional vitality in every bite

2. Full enzyme potency while preserving your own diminished enzyme bank account

3. Optimal intestinal absorption

Is it any wonder that our Birchcreek program gets the finest results anywhere? You can solve the two major causes of obesity and disease—deficiency and toxicity—by eating high-octane living food filled with naturally occurring detoxifiers. This provides a double-barreled approach that affords you the most rapid, safe weight loss you can possibly achieve, plus a restoration of health and vitality.

In the back of this book you will find Birchcreek's Ten-Juice Fast program for rapid, healthy weight loss and detoxification, as well as plenty of delicious recipes.

CHAPTER 8

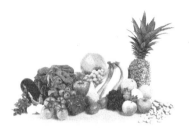

CHARTING A NEW COURSE

If you ask the same old questions you will get the same old answers. If you ask different questions...you will get different answers.

In order to realize what you can achieve, you must stop allowing yourself to be bound by old wives' tales and outdated paradigms. A paradigm is a model of understanding, and paradigms can be very hard to change. Your paradigms and beliefs have been seeded by what you have heard and read and by the people of influence in your life. All of us assemble these ideas and bits of information into a belief system or a paradigm by which we operate. We simply believe what we believe to be true. This is truth for us.

Even though other people have created for themselves different paradigms, ours prevails for us, and we conduct our lives by it. Can anyone be completely right—or completely wrong? In all probability most of us are somewhat right and somewhat wrong. Shouldn't we want to get closer to the absolute truth? To do that, perhaps we should require better answers to the questions we have about what's true.

If we expect to make lasting, permanent changes in our weight, health, and well-being, we need better answers to the same old questions. After all, most people purchase a book like this because they are looking for better answers than they have already. They have come to the inevitable conclusion that diets don't work, at least the ones they have tried.

Perhaps you tell people that you have tried every diet known to man. By now you know that there are no silver bullet diets. Regardless of whether or not you have high hopes as you read this book, you've made the right choice. We are prepared to answer some perplexing questions.

BETTER ANSWERS TO THE SAME OLD QUESTIONS

Let's start with some of the major concerns people have about dieting: "Will I be hungry?" "What about the taste of the food on this diet?" "What about meat and dairy?" "What about protein?" "Oh yes, and how much weight can I lose, and how fast should I lose it?" One question I really love to answer is this: "Is fish meat?" I have a whimsical way of answering that (forgive me). I tell people, "If it has eyes or a rear end, it is meat."

For our purposes the meat questions are the big ones. I fully understand people's reluctance to abandon meat in their diets. The truth is, *there is not one nutritional advantage to consuming meat that can't be met abundantly with a plant-based diet, including adequate protein.*

If the answer to the dilemma of eating cooked food is to eat raw food, what about raw fish? I would say if you trust your source of your raw fish, go ahead and eat it! I wouldn't take a chance on the bacteria that you might ingest if you eat fish that has not been handled carefully. But if you trust your source, go ahead and add it to your diet, because when you eat it, you will be getting a full complement of enzymes and a safe amount of bacteria to help with its rapid digestion. I think about the Eskimos, who originally lived on raw blubber and raw mackerel and whose society showed an extremely low incidence of heart disease and diabetes.

Almost universally, raw food, regardless of what it is, is better than cooked food. In an agrarian Asian culture, a family would sit around a table and share an abundance of vegetables and fruit. In the middle of that table would be the delicacy— a small piece of meat. The quantity of meat would be only about the size of your hand, and yet it would feed five or more members of the family. Each person would get a narrow sliver of meat as a delicacy. Many times the meat would have been naturally cured. There is a big difference between that and a quarter-pounder per person per day!

MY ICON, MY UNCLE

My uncle Angelo lived to a pretty ripe old age. He was hardly sick a day in his life. He was really amazing. When he finally passed away, he was in the best shape I had ever seen for a person his age. He lived a full, healthy life. In fact, he was aggressive in his love for life.

He told me, "I rarely go to a doctor, but when I do, the first thing I ask a doctor is, 'What number did you graduate in your class?'" He wanted to make sure that his doctor had finished first, second, or third in the graduating class. I don't know if I possess the nerve to ask such a question. He told me that he wouldn't even go to a doctor unless that doctor was technically capable. Also, he insisted on speaking with the doctor for as long as he would be tolerated. At some point the doctor would say to him, "Listen, I have other patients, and I can't just hang out all day and chat with you."

Uncle Angelo would reply, "But I need to know a little bit more about you if you're going to know more about me." When I asked him what he meant by that, he said, "I had to find out if this guy had common sense. What good would he be to me if he couldn't use his brain to find the obvious?"

Maybe you have had these same thoughts. You walk into a doctor's office with an ailment, a pain. He checks you out and diagnoses the problem. He was trained to diagnosis problems, and he is an expert in his field. Then what does he do? He consults his expertise in the use of medicines that can be prescribed for different ailments. Now what just happened? He is not applying common sense, but rather he is simply applying protocol. The remedy is a medicine. The protocol is driven by expedience. The fact is, if the medical field would just apply a little common sense to identify the root causes of various ailments, they would use less medicine.

Some medical experts do just that, and we can learn a lot from them.

LOOK TOWARD THE EXPERTS

Doctors Joel Fuhrman, who specializes in nutritional treatments for obesity and chronic diseases such as heart disease, and Neal Barnard, who is the founder and president of the Physicians Committee for Responsible Medicine, have both been on the leading edge of research in the fields of diet and health. In their many papers and books they agree that the root cause of premature death is our reliance on meat, dairy, and cooked food, and that this reliance leads to our biggest killers: heart disease, cancer, and diabetes. The numbers would be even more alarming if the percentages of unnecessary premature deaths due to various causes, such as kidney failure, were blamed on the underlying cause of chronic heart disease. Because the heart is the primary functioning organ that regulates other organs on many levels, the health and effectiveness of the kidneys may be the smoking gun while the root cause may be a weak or damaged heart.

We read the statistics that 54 percent of unnecessary premature deaths are due initially to heart disease, while 38 percent of the population will die of cancer.[1] If you eliminate cigarette smoking, you would almost totally eliminate lung cancer except for those incidents of contact with agitators such as asbestos and other caustic ingested poisons or carcinogens. Death from any other cause is at 8 percent, which includes diabetes, arthritis, Alzheimer's disease, degenerative, digestive, and immune disorders.[2] In addition, the American Medical Association has indicated that unnecessary hospital deaths total an average of 225,000 a year. Such deaths occur from misdiagnosis, misappropriation of medications, incorrect dosages of medications, and incidences of staph infections.[3]

NATURAL CAUSES

The medical profession is doing all they can to control this epidemic of unnatural death. Is there anyone out there dying of "natural causes" anymore? I would define death by natural causes as a person living into his early to midnineties with minimal medical intervention, who, active and useful one day, turns in for the night and doesn't awaken the next day. I would define an unnatural death as living the last ten to fifteen years of life in poor and failing health, dependent on an endless stream of meds, worsening day by day for years, and spending the last five years of life in and out of hospitals. We seem to be defining natural causes differently these days. Recently a celebrity died from "natural causes" although she was on prescription medications and her death really was a result of a drug overdose. I would rather die of ripe old age, wouldn't you?

Vegans (those who do not consume animal products and who eat a strictly plant-based diet) have been included in these statistics for unnecessary premature death. Just think—without vegans being included in that equation, those statistics would be horrifically higher. Over the past twenty-five years surveys show that people who are living on plant-based diets suffer far less from heart disease and cancers. In addition, diabetes, arthritis, and osteoporosis occur so much less often that the medical profession should have taken notice.[4]

Congress is beginning to take notice and is pushing to create boundaries, restrictions, rules, regulations, and qualifications for health and weight-loss retreats. Why do you think they have become so interested in nonclinical approaches to weight loss and detoxification? I conjecture that it has something to do with dollar signs.

For my part I want to give my body every opportunity to perform as it was designed, and that includes fueling it with the right foods. Of course the physical differences between us will always exist, but our genes are not in total control over what ails us. I reiterate: heredity is not a ticking time bomb.

These days obesity is considered a disease often driven by heredity. Is obesity something that might befall someone whose luck runs out or who has angered some cosmic force? I doubt it.

Life is a choice, not a chancy proposition that is out of your control. What choices can you start making *today* to lengthen and improve your life? At the end of your allotted time on earth, I am sure that you want to be among those who die with dignity and of natural causes.

CHAPTER 9

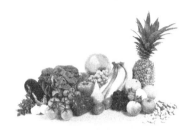

THE SMART BODY

Your body is smart; it runs on automatic pilot, prede-signed, already calibrated, and ready to go. Designed with incredible intricacy and a high order of operation, sustaining health and correcting problems as they arise, the functions of the human body are almost miraculous.

Your body conducts millions upon millions of operations every second you are alive. The autonomic characteristic of your body, the part that is on automatic pilot, makes up more than 99 percent of your bodily functions. You and I are only in charge of operating less than 1 percent of our bodily functions, if that many.

It is as if we come equipped with an "operating system," just like a laptop computer. On that system we can find all our autonomic and somatic functions. There are programs for cell division; for blood-clotting; for regulating body temperature, heart rate, blood pressure, and the production of hormones— just to name a few. Meanwhile all we are aware of doing is walking around, taking a drink, going to the bathroom, making babies, making war, and making excuses (pardon the cynicism). This autonomic system is a remote control system, unlike the somatic system, which is activated and controlled by our conscience minds.

Our autonomic systems have been programmed from birth. Our somatic systems must be programmed by means of what we learn, our personalities, and our willful responses to outside stimuli. As we grow up, we get introduced to many stimuli, which include many sensations such as touch, taste, feel, and smell. They became the macros in our programming, and we respond without hesitation or evaluation much of the time.

A lifetime of chemical introductions, poor nutrition, and toxicity serve to corrupt our autonomic programs much as a virus corrupts a computer program. As the program becomes corrupted, it begins to malfunction. Just as a computer virus permeates our operating system's ability to deal with normal routines, so it is with our biology. Garbage in yields garbage out. We are asking our operating system to do things it was never designed to do and to deal with conditions it was not designed to deal with.

WOMB TO TOMB

Exploring the inner workings of our incredible, smart body starts at the beginning, with life from prebirth. Before birth every one of us was hooked to our mother's blood supply by an umbilical cord. This blood supply carried with it all the nutrition required for rapid growth. From one cell at conception, we became 75 trillion cells by the time of birth. For up to three to six months after birth we added new cells, reaching 100 trillion total cells upon completion.

Even if a mother isn't taking care of herself, the baby gets everything he needs at mom's expense, except for in the most extreme cases of prenatal malnutrition. Because we have all of our nutritional needs met so thoroughly, it is as if we become preprogrammed for good nutrition. In the last trimester of growth inside the mother the baby is growing in leaps and bounds. The drain on the mother's nutritional system is incredible. If she is not careful, she may begin to show signs of nutrition deficiency such as skin disorders or fragile nails, hair, and teeth. All the nutrition is going to that little baby. That baby is hooked up to mommy and needs nothing but a nice, warm, cozy place to grow. For the most part all of his nutritional needs are being met.

As that baby grows and gets nearer to the time of birth, she shifts and turns and gets ready to start moving down the birth canal. The process of labor begins. During delivery a baby encounters physiological tension as she begins to squeeze through the birth canal. The infant's entire history at this point consists of the minimal sensations of being in the mother's womb for nine months. After birth the baby's physical tension is quelled by washing, cuddling, and being wrapped in soft blankets to simulate the womb environment. Bodily functions that were dormant just a moment ago start to work. Air is breathed for the first time, as if a switch has been flipped. It is a whole new world with new sensations. Miraculously the baby's entire physiology has been preprogrammed to start and run for the first time just moments after birth.

When the umbilical cord gets cut at birth, the baby's brain registers an interruption in the flow of nutrition. That baby has been filled and overflowing with nutrition for nine months. But when that first minute of interruption sends that baby into a physiological panic anxiety, what is done to alleviate that anxiety? Put her on mommy's breast, and almost instantly that baby starts to suckle. The miraculous construction of the baby's mouth and the receptors on that baby's tongue communicate to the brain and to the operating system, "OK, we've recovered our nutrition." Now the baby is using different faculties. She never needed her mouth to eat before. But with the proverbial slap on the bottom, this baby is performing like the rest of us. The remarkable part of this bodily function is that when the baby's tongue comes into contact with even a few drops of her mother's colostrum or milk, it recognizes nutrition and sends a message to the brain.

ADDICTED TO NUTRITION

You can safely say that from birth you have been addicted to nutrition. The needs of your body are satisfied by nutrition. As you grow, you begin to spread your wings. When you can hold your head up, mommy weans you from breast milk to other forms of nutrition. Often and early on you got introduced to nutritional imposters, substances that were processed from sources of true nutrition to resemble the tastes they represent—with processed sugar and processed salt leading the pack.

Watch a baby's eyes and expression to clearly see the response when experiencing a taste other than milk for the first time. Some parents put sugar or something sweet on baby's tongue and watch as the baby responds accordingly. Almost all babies gravitate to and love sugary sweet tastes and recoil in shivered horror to bitter or sour tastes, spitting out the spinach and all the other stuff that doesn't taste as sweet as applesauce or honey.

Is it as simple as this little baby liking or disliking the particular tastes of particular foods, or is there something more profound afoot? As the tongue contains receptors that receive and transmit to the operating system what is passing through the mouth and heading toward the rest of the digestive system, that baby's autonomic system is in full operation on the most discreet of levels.

Sugar placed on the tongue actually tricks the brain by registering on its receptor cells as glucose (the fundamental food source for every cell in the body). Coincidentally, bitter and sour tastes resemble acidic food substances, which are, from a biological point of view, the body's archenemies. If a receptor cell senses acidity, the brain responds, "How dare you do such a thing to me? Why did you put this poison in my mouth?" Thus we have a natural affinity to sweets and an aversion toward bitter and sour things. If you were seriously dehydrated, you might find yourself in a hospital on an intravenous infusion. If you tasted what was in the bag of that intravenous drip, you'd find glucose water tasting sweet, just like sugar. That inborn preference remains the same for life, although we can "hack into" it and send it false data.

TASTE COMES FIRST

I was born into an Italian household. My mother was well educated in the art of feeding her children. She was always worried about her "little Ronnie" having enough food. When my mother passed away, my oldest daughter made me a collage of about a dozen or so pictures of my mom and me from age six to twenty-one. Every single picture showed my mother following me around with a bowl of food. Mothers all over the world worry about their baby's health and well-being. Somehow babies save the day and let moms know that to save their precious lives, they need applesauce or pears or some other sweet-tasting food to rescue them. Even carrots can pass the taste test as long as it is in the sweet family. Is it any wonder why we gravitate toward sweets? Our moms are steadily and surely being conditioned to feed their "little Ronnies" what they will agree to eat. Mommy doesn't realize that she has been manipulated so she will serve exactly what passes the taste test with little regard for nutrition. Thank God for fruit. How many little children would perish? Or would they?

When we become old enough to choose our own breakfast or lunch, we naturally gravitate toward what is dictated by our tastes. As a teenager I would go to the Italian deli and get a large hero sandwich of crusty Italian bread covered with sesame seeds and stuffed with salami, Swiss cheese, tomato, and mustard. I'd wash it down with a quart of Coke. That was my lunch, and I loved it. I couldn't have cared less about nutrition.

But I was addicted to it. Like everyone else I was addicted to carbohydrates, fats, proteins, and glucose. The consequence of withdrawal from carbohydrates, fats, proteins, and glucose is starvation. And total starvation is death. You see, you can't do without nutrition. You can do without any other addiction, but not this one. Withdrawal from food is called hunger. Actually, hunger is the symptom associated when withdrawing from anything addictive. Withdrawal symptoms create a physiological anxiety, whether the withdrawal is from nicotine, caffeine, alcohol, or nutrition. Withdrawal from addictive drugs will cause physiological anxiety. But with food a complete withdrawal causes death.

When my body is hungry, it craves nutrition. To quench that hunger, I look for food. It doesn't take long for an infant to recognize that every time he shows a little anxiety for food, mommy is right there to supply it. The severe peak of anxiety is diminished by the repetition of the remedy. So from infancy we have developed a habit of quenching our anxiety with food.

And not just any old food will do. When we go to a restaurant and open a menu, do we look only for something that is good for us? That would be abnormal since by the time we are young adults, we have successfully supplanted the inborn need for nutrition with our learned desire for taste.

Our operating system, like Microsoft Windows, is telling us nutrition is needed. The programs we have installed on our operating system are designed to satisfy our prime directive, the acquiring of nutrition for survival. Our body's autonomic system will jump through hoops to correct the lack of proper fuel, but we all manage to corrupt the perfect program we were designed with. Having been schooled in taste, we consume foods that offer the most superficial satisfaction. Early in life our somatic system has been reprogrammed, like Pavlov's dog. We have been conditioned to use an implanted connection to nutrition, *our taste.* We are now driven by a poor substitute for nutritional gratification, namely processed imposters, sugar and salt. We gravitate toward processed sugar and processed salt (which impersonate glucose and sodium).

You walk into the movie theater and smell popcorn and begin to salivate. You crave food because you like what it tastes like, and it stimulates the process of digestion without your even tasting it. It may or may not have a connection to nutrition at all. You fool your operating system for a short while. Then you're hungry again, and the cycle repeats itself. You've created a trigger with every TV commercial you watch and every fast-food billboard you see, because they stimulate your basic need for nutrition, now driven almost solely by taste. (There's an irony in fast foods. Fast-food restaurants add food to both of your primary trigger mechanisms: processed sugar and salt.)

In its processed form salt is like poison to your body. Salt as sodium is an essential element you need to derive from food. Your body doesn't produce it. But when it has been processed rather than being naturally derived from plant foods, your body wants to get rid of it. If processed salt enters your body, your autonomic system begins to diminish the effect of the salt in a most ingenious way: your body begins to retain water for the sole purpose of diluting that poison. Your smart body is at work against this poison, trying desperately to alleviate its damaging effects on your health.

Yet many people persist in going to restaurants that add sugar, salt, and variations of other tastes to foods, which artificially raises the threshold of satisfaction. All is not lost, because you can retrain your tastes. That's what we help people do at Birchcreek, and we are about to tell you how to do it in this book.

RESENSITIZING YOUR TASTE BUDS

At Birchcreek we prove a point through a test. We prove to people that they can truly enjoy the taste of natural foods again. We put people on a detoxing juice fast for one week. After that time period they taste a fruit, vegetable, or healthy snack that they didn't used to think was salty or sweet enough in its natural form. This time they can't believe how tasty it is! They are surprised how salty or how sweet something can naturally be once they have detoxed and returned sensitivity to their taste buds. They may be experiencing and enjoying natural fructose and natural sodium in raw foods for the first time ever. The aromas, textures, and flavors explode, and surprise is hard to subdue! Invariably they are satisfied beyond their expectations. Their brains begin to reprogram themselves.

Still, our volition, our somatic system, always attempts to supersede our taste-driven autonomic system. Hunger can be a painful experience. As humans we not only resist hunger at all costs, but we also fortify ourselves against the sensation of hunger by eating enough to last to our next meal. Our body chemistry is a result of not only the food we eat but also our social habits. If we smoke and drink, we already know that these things are not good for the chemistry of our bodies. Most states have now banned smoking in public places because of societal awareness of this fact. Our physical environment can lead to poor body chemistry. If we live in a smog-ridden city, if we are sucking down bus fumes all the time, or if we are traveling in subways all the time, our body chemistry suffers.

All these things trigger an autonomic response in our systems to correct and adjust for maximum efficiency and immediate preservation of life.

Weight gain is one of the primary indicators of poor health. Too many people come to our retreat claiming they really eat healthy foods, yet for some reason they are sixty pounds or more overweight. In fact, it is that "good food" they *think* they are eating that is killing them slowly, and their bodies cannot compensate for the deficiencies indefinitely.

The food we eat gets utilized in two ways: short-term readily available use and long-term use. Short-term energy foods get converted into glucose for rapid, readily available burnable fuel for the machine. Long-term fuel is stored for use at a later time. It is being conserved for a rainy day or for an emergency. The standard American diet is almost entirely composed of foods (in the form of fats and processed carbohydrates) that are meant for long-term use. These potential fuels are most often converted into fat cells first. Fat cells, of course, contain potential fuel, which can later be converted into high-octane fuel (glucose) if and when needed. The problem is that the fatter we get, the more lethargic we become. And the more lethargic we become, the less likely we are to summon those fat reserves for the conversion process.

Ask yourself a question: Are you eating short-term energy foods, or are you eating foods better designed for fat storage for a later date? Some foods are well designed to release energy slowly and on demand. Athletes often eat pasta or grains before an event in order to have a "top end," a late and lasting burst of sustained energy toward the end of the competition. This is a forced conversion. Without converting this unused carbohydrate into glucose, it remains as stored fat. Are you eating foods that are suited as long-term fat stores for an emergency? Or are you eating foods that are suited for being converted into energy first with only the unused energy stored as fat (such as grains, beans, legumes, seeds, and nuts)?

You see, without energy you will never have the ability to burn calories. Without burning the calories you are eating, you tend to convert all calories into fat. These types of foods have an almost impossible task of starting off as easily burn-able fuel: french fries, hamburgers and steak, cold cuts and breads, packaged and processed foods, and the like. These foods store fat first, and the potential energy is only released if you have the constitution to work out two hours a day.

Why do Americans have a hard time exercising? If you were to ask sedentary people why they don't exercise, you'd get the same answer over and over again: "I don't have the time." The actual reason is because they don't have *the energy* to exercise. The foods Americans eat are low-octane, highly inefficient, fat-storing, high-calorie, and high waste-producing foods.

TIME TO REBOOT

How much energy do you have? If you were able to measure your vitality, the spring in your step, the strength of your tendons and ligaments, or the efficiency of your organs and then compare them to how they should be, you might be frightened into making big changes in your eating. Instead, most of us just measure health by hopping on a scale. We look at our weight and declare, "I've got to lose weight." And what is our method to lose this weight? We begin to count calories. We start to measure our food, weigh or measure carbohydrates, or weigh the amount of protein we are consuming. The problem is that although those things will cause weight loss, they are merely a cosmetic fix. It is micromanaging the most basic instinct, which is the instinct to eat. Meanwhile starvation is stifling your need for nutrition. When we micromanage an already poor diet, we are left in a more precarious condition, and we put our bodies into a state of constant emergency.

If we institute no significant change in nutrition, our internal programming has no options for change. You have to install a different program on your operating system, your restored autonomic system, fueled and maintained into old age with proper foods. Your autonomic system is like a computer. When your computer begins to labor, get sticky, and become loaded with junk, when it is no longer as agile as it was when it was new and it doesn't get around as quickly, we reboot that system. Rebooting might mean shutting it off and putting it back on, or it might mean taking off all the programs so you can start over.

The Birchcreek Jump-Start Your Life program reboots your operating system with detoxification. By detoxifying, we are decontaminating the operating system that was preoccupied with trying to put out fires from programs that were corrupted. By detoxifying, we are purifying the environment. Now because the environment in our retreat setting doesn't have the smell of popcorn, steak, or rack of lamb (or the draw from social activities that contaminate our chemistry), we are literally taking those corrupted programs and putting them on the side. Remember these are just programs. They are not necessary and can be replaced.

The next thing we might do for our computer is to install

virus protection, right? In a similar way the Birchcreek Jump-Start Your Life program is also virus protection. It consists of knowledge, understanding, and, hopefully, wisdom. Even though clients are ultimately responsible to apply their reasoning and common sense to what we teach, we supply logical instructions to make success easier. When you come to Birchcreek, there are only two things required. Participate in all we offer, and get out of your own way. Take your belief system, your model of understanding that you came with, and allow us to give you a new model of understanding and a new base of knowledge. We will do our best to add understanding to that knowledge so that you can begin to implement knowledge in programs and changes that will benefit your life and your longevity.

The wisdom component comes when you implement the knowledge and understanding correctly. If you have wisdom, you can use your knowledge, and you will be able to discern the landscape before you get there. You will need to know how to negotiate around what is dangerously bad for you and how to find what is good for you; that ability to discern is the "virus protection" that Birchcreek offers.

You know that when you buy virus protection for your computer, you still have the freedom to make good or bad choices. Even with good virus protection installed on your new computer, you will sometimes get alert warnings: "If you open this program, it could be damaging to your system." Even though you have the virus protection, you still have to make the right decisions.

When knowledge and understanding come along, you are able to execute wisdom. You have to live with your convictions and decisions—right, wrong, or indifferent. Sometimes you will make the wrong decision, because you are not perfect and you don't always do the right thing. I don't know anyone who leaves our program with a halo and little angel wings. We all have the ability to make poor choices, and we often do, but that is no disqualification for attending the Birchcreek program.

A POWERFUL INSURANCE POLICY

If you are living a life that is being fueled with proper nutrition, and every now and then you eat something that you know is not very good for you, your body will be well equipped to handle it. The occasional poor choice is not the problem. But how can you be sure you will stay on track? Can you get some kind of an insurance policy?

Birchcreek offers one in the form of the Stay on Track program. This insurance policy insures nearly 100 percent success because people who join this program are engaging in accountability. Accountability means that we can walk together down this road while using the Jump-Start Your Life program and the Stay on Track program. (See more information about our Stay on Track program on our website at www .weightlossretreat.com.)

Together is the operative word. We understand the problems, pitfalls, and situations that confound you. The Stay on Track program works as a referee that breaks the unhealthy cycles and encourages you. You are never too late; you are never too sick to start where you are and take the next step. The program will coach, mentor, and encourage you. It is easy to see the difference between the people who have someone to walk alongside and those walking alone.

We encourage everyone to join the Stay on Track program. The program works because of the ease and efficiency of electronic media communication. It is powerful and effective. We have the ability to conduct roundtable discussions and webinars every month. People who join the Stay on Track program can share our seminars with loved ones. You can receive the help you need to move forward with staying power and to show others firsthand evidence of your success.

CHAPTER 10

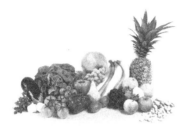

STRATEGIZING FOR SUCCESS

I t is our hope that this book will be a powerful tool to transform communities around the country. As your health and fitness reach dramatic improvement, your family and friends will want to know what you are doing to create such obvious changes. Your example will influence your whole social community and even those you have yet to meet on this new adventure.

The only way to succeed at maintaining a healthy lifestyle is to find ways that will work to motivate you personally to sustain the changes you have made in your eating patterns. Picture a sturdy, rock-solid tripod. The three legs have these words etched on them: Biology, Strategy, and Support.

BIOLOGY

This truth pertains to your biological well-being, and it remains true whether or not you believe it. Your body functions at its best only if you make the right choices. Your biology depends on you to make right choices. In the beginning some people are so determined to change, only to find out that they are ruled by the cravings for all the foods they have come to love. They find themselves slaves to their urges and cravings; they are in the middle of a war between truth and their taste buds. When their taste buds try to control their willpower, which used to win, they need to remind themselves that they possess new truth, knowledge, and understanding. They have to remember how their bodies responded during that first miraculous week of the Birchcreek program, when their cravings and runaway hunger were quenched through high-octane, great-tasting juices and raw foods.

The battle of your will is not as challenging as you might think. Success is sweet, and your unexpected vitality and weight loss propel you forward. Success is easy because you are beginning to meet your body's nutritional requirements perhaps as never before. It is not a stretch of the truth to state that a body completely nutritionally satiated will become very content.

I encourage everyone to take a week and detoxify by juicing. The phrase *juice fast* has a connotation of deprivation or sacrifice. Clients who come to Birchcreek receive juices made from 8 to 9 pounds of produce a day. It wouldn't be possible to eat that much. The juice they drink is equivalent to six times more quality nutrition than the average overweight, undernourished American eats on a daily basis. After one to one and a half days of detoxifying (detox), your hunger will disappear. Your autonomic system will be telling you, "I'm overwhelmed with nutrition, I have no hunger triggers, and I am keeping myself safe. And I'm not hungry."

STRATEGY

The purpose of starting is to finish. You are now in new territory. Continuing a lifestyle change is not the same as a weekly retreat. You cannot expect to live exclusively on juices beyond one or two weeks. You need strategies to create the transition from one lifestyle to another. You have the truth, you have the will to change, and it is time to put truth into action.

Now you need to keep priming the machine until it stays started. You can use your body's own autonomic tendencies to correct your poor eating habits. On top of your previous autonomic tendencies, the tendencies that were susceptible to your old eating habits, you are now going to superimpose new habits, good habits. Remember, it is not so much about will-power as it is about reprogramming.

Creatures of habit, we crave what we already eat. And we rely on those easily recognizable triggers, like taste, to build our cravings. Why not broaden your repertoire? If you can begin to satisfy your taste with what you know your autonomic system needs, high-octane living foods, you can retrain your cravings.

The process must not be difficult. Choose foods that are wholesome, that are right for the biology of your body, and that *taste good*. It is not possible to change if you think you are going to be forced to eat tasteless or bad-tasting foods. Find a good combination between raw and cooked foods, and choose foods that are high in octane, low in waste, and that taste great. It should go without saying that you should choose foods that are accessible to you. You need to be able to purchase your foods in the average supermarket.

SUPPORT

People who successfully break habits and addictions must be connected to some type of support system. Nobody can sustain success without one. As I mentioned in the previous chapter, Birchcreek has a wonderful and highly effective alumni support program that is appropriately named Stay on Track. For people who have not participated in our retreat program, we have a powerful and easy-to-follow Get on Track program.

All of our support programs follow the same three-step template while containing personalized strategies that are highly effective. Both the Stay on Track and the Get on Track programs are unique, like having your own tutor!

But how can you maintain the new, trim you? By micromanaging your whole life for the rest of your life? None of us can sustain antiquated methods such as weighing food or counting calories, carbohydrates, protein, or fats.

As time goes by, your resolve slips. The very first time you miss a week of activity, you begin to regain weight quickly. Weight and fat begin to accumulate faster than you can exercise it off or metabolize it. Eventually and assuredly you cannot permanently micromanage your dietary life. Why not? Because your body feels unnaturally and nutritionally deprived.

We were designed to consume natural foods. When we

practice eating natural foods, we recalibrate our systems naturally and permanently.

Follow this simple three-step, easy-to-remember TOA rule:

1. Taste: Do not deprive your taste buds.

2. Octane: Eat food high in octane (more living, raw food).

3. Access: Select foods you can get at your local supermarket.

Understand that the height of the physiological anxiety caused by the apparent deprivation or withdrawal from nutrition has an interesting correlation to the satisfaction gained when we quench that condition. No one who hungers for fruits and vegetables receives such tremendous satisfaction from their consumption as from processed or highly prepared foods. Consuming fruits and vegetables never creates peaks and valleys. Only by artificially treating food to satisfy our tastes will we get the kinds of satisfaction we get when we go to a great restaurant. We begin to anticipate and desire restaurant and processed foods because they have been engineered so that even if we are not hungry, they will satisfy us far more than any fruit or vegetable ever can.

The solution is to detoxify to raise the sensitivity of your taste buds so you can appreciate the variety of tastes, textures, and aromas in plant-based foods.

If I were to invite you to dinner tomorrow evening at your favorite restaurant where they make your favorite food (and you do not have the opportunity to eat that food very often), it is likely that when you get up in the morning, you'll be anticipating the upcoming dinner. About midmorning you'll start thinking, "I don't want to eat anything because I don't want to spoil my appetite before tonight's dinner." What you are really doing is raising your physiological anxiety in order to derive more pleasure from the food you were waiting for. Normally hunger is an unpleasant sensation, and we try to prevent it at all costs. But remember, the height of physiological anxiety is equal to the measure of satisfaction when food finally touches your tongue. If we make a habit of operating this way, this habit feeds into an already bad program. It is like adding corrupted information to an already corrupted operating system. We must allow our autonomic system to help us change those corrupted programs into clean, valuable, and efficient programs. It won't happen as long as we keep sending ourselves the equivalent of e-mail spam!

After accepting the concept of working with your physiology instead of against it, you come to terms with your own resolve. Suddenly the mystery of losing and keeping unwanted weight off becomes a reality. Understanding what makes you tick, so to speak, becomes the strategy. Within the three requirements—biology, strategy, and support—we find ourselves ready, willing, and able to advance into success. Working with your body instead of fighting against it makes you far wiser in your approach than most, if not all, other diet plans. There are no shortcuts, but there is a clearly marked road map that is easily traveled.

CHAPTER 11

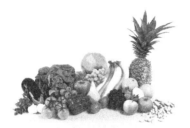

DON'T PHOOL WITH YOUR PH

At Birchcreek, new guests are often proud of the fact that they had their pH tested and the results were "perfect." But what do most people know about pH? Is pH an indicator of overall health? Is 7, 7.1, 7.2, or 7.25 a good reading for blood pH? What is the significance of small increments between these numbers?

These pH measurements reflect the chemistry of the body relative to the balance between acidity and alkalinity in the blood. Acid is a by-product or an end product of metabolism from energy production. Alkalinity results from the metabolism of calcium. Both acidity and alkalinity can be measured by using blood pH, saliva pH, or urine pH. (A blood pH is a more reliable and stable reading of body chemistry, since saliva and urine are easily affected by recent food consumption.)

For our purposes we will be referring to blood pH. A good blood pH number is 7.35, which is slightly alkaline. Anything lower than that is veering toward the acidic end, and the more acidic the pH, the more sickness or poor health is indicated.

RELATIVE pH OF COMMON SUBSTANCES

Eating high-energy, high-octane food produces less waste and results in less acidity. When people are young, their immune systems have the ability to quickly and efficiently remove this waste and neutralize acidity. But nobody stays young forever. Time, wear, and tear are great equalizers. After a period of time the body begins to lose the ability to adjust its chemistry when the diet has consisted of so many foods that create acidity.

ENTER... YOUR SMART BODY

The autonomic system begins to use an array of fail-safe programs and responses to maintain the required 7.35 blood pH that will maintain life within the range of good health. However, it can only achieve balance for so long before it begins to falter. We need to feed our bodies to help keep them balanced.

Certain foods naturally produce acid, while other foods create conditions of acidity. The metabolizing of animal protein produces acid, and animal products also produce an overpopulation of harmful bacteria in the gut. Animal products tend to stick around in our system much too long, and they begin to putrefy. This decomposition serves as perfect nourishment for these harmful bacteria that proliferate, producing their own waste, which consists of almost pure acid. Now an acid emergency exists in the body.

After the immune system can no longer maintain a clean chemistry, there are two specific protocols the autonomic system incorporates to maintain cleanliness and a proper pH. For the most part these emergency protocols go unnoticed, although they do not take place without certain evidence. For example, when a person begins to gain weight, when cholesterol levels increase, when sugar (blood glucose) goes up, when blood pressure becomes elevated, when joints ache, when sleep quality becomes poor, when acid reflux develops, and so on—all these are signs that a person needs to make a course correction.

The person who has eaten a tremendous amount of cooked food, meat, and dairy for a number of years will have at least two emergency responses poised for intervention if they are not already intervening. That person's body is in imminent danger; it is in survival mode. If, on the other hand, a person concentrates heavily on fruits and vegetables and a lot of raw food, that person's system will have a naturally occurring pH of close to 7.35, and the autonomic system will be able to operate in a business-as-usual manner.

THE MISER

The most prevalent way your autonomic system saves your life on a daily basis is by initiating the emergency response that I call the "miser protocol." While saving your life today, the miser protocol does not take into account the far-reaching consequences to your life in years to come. Here's how the miser protocol works.

As acid molecules attack muscle and organ tissue and especially that of the most vital organ, your heart, your body begins to hoard fat. Instead of using food as energy, it starts storing it as fat. Fat can only be transformed into energy if you exercise, and the fatter you become, the less energy you have for that.

What is the purpose of the extra fat stores? The miser protocol stores fat for the sole purpose of leeching serum cholesterol into the blood to bind acid. Binding the acid molecules renders them impotent so they can no longer do damage to your organs. It is an amazing emergency response. Just as during hypothermia your blood shifts to vital organs to save your life, your autonomic system doesn't consider the consequences of clogged arteries from coagulated serum cholesterol ten years from now when you enter an emergency acidic blood state. It is functioning to keep you alive second by second and for the next 365 days.

We all know someone who seems to be able to eat anything, as much and as often as they like, without gaining weight. We assume that these people are healthier than those who are overweight or gain weight easily. Yet often such people die from the same conditions (heart disease or stroke) as heavier people. Your friend may be thin on the outside but fat on the inside.

THE THIEF

Even if this system is like Robin Hood, stealing from the rich to give to the poor, a thief is still a thief, and there are consequences to the act of keeping a person alive during an acid emergency. The thief also leaves behind destruction and desolation.

For instance, your body will steal calcium in order to maintain proper pH. And it will not ask your permission to do so. If you are eating foods that are not high in metabolically absorbable calcium (which would be living food containing active enzymes to help with the metabolism of the calcium), you will not be getting the by-product of this process, which is alkaline ash, the counterbalance against acid. To make up for the lack, your body looks around, notices your wonderful, living, calcium-rich skeleton, and says, "Wow, I have all the calcium I will ever need." The autonomic system begins to deplete and digest its own skeleton for the purpose of creating an alkaline ash to balance the overabundance of acid in your body that was caused by an acid-producing diet of meat and dairy foods.

The results are predictable: osteoporosis, primarily. This is another example of the way we can trace debilitating disorders to something as basic as our diet.

WHAT TO EAT

Some foods that seem acidic are actually alkaline-forming. To avoid confusion, refer to the following charts summarizing foods to avoid (acid-forming) and foods to frequent (alkaline-forming). You can find more complete lists online if you are interested in looking up a particular food or in rebalancing your diet. Note that many plant foods that are slightly acid-producing, such as legumes, are so beneficial that they are certainly worth eating when combined with an overall alkaline diet.

ALKALINE-FORMING FOODS	
VEGETABLES	Alfalfa · Asparagus · Barley grass · Beets · Broccoli · Brussels sprouts · Cabbage · Carrots · Cauliflower · Celery · Chard · Chlorella · Collard · Cucumber · Dandelions · Dulce · Eggplant · Fermented vegetables · Garlic · Kale · Kohlrabi · Lettuce · Mushrooms · Mustard greens · Nightshade vegetables · Onions · Parsnips · Peas · Peppers · Pumpkin · Rutabaga · Sea vegetables · Spirulina · Sprouts · Squashes · Watercress · Wheatgrass
FRUITS	Apples · Apricots · Avocados · Bananas · Berries · Cantaloupe · Cherries · Currants · Dates/figs · Grapefruit · Grapes · Honeydew · Lemons · Limes · Nectarines · Oranges · Peaches · Pears · Pineapple · Tangerines · Tomatoes · Tropical fruits · Watermelon
PROTEIN	Almonds · Chestnuts · Flaxseeds · Millet · Nuts · Pumpkin seeds · Sprouted seeds · Squash seeds · Tempeh · Tofu · Yogurt
MISCELLANEOUS FOODS	All herbs · Apple cider vinegar · Bee pollen · Chili pepper · Cinnamon · Curry · Daikon · Dandelion root · Fresh fruit juices · Ginger · Green juices · Kombu · Kombucha · Lecithin granules · Maitake · Mineral water · Miso · Mustard · Nori · Organic milk (unpasteurized) · Probiotic cultures · Reishi · Sea salt · Shiitake · Stevia · Tamari · Umeboshi · Vegetable juices · Wakame

ACID-FORMING FOODS	
FATS AND OILS	Avocado oil · Canola oil · Corn oil · Flax oil · Hemp seed oil · Lard · Olive oil · Safflower oil · Sesame oil · Sunflower oil
FRUITS	Cranberries
GRAINS	Amaranth · Barley · Buckwheat · Corn · Hemp seed flour · Kamut · Oats · Quinoa · Rice (all types) · Rye · Spelt · Wheat
DAIRY	All cheeses · Almond milk · Butter · Milk · Rice milk · Soy milk
NUTS AND NUT BUTTERS	Brazil nuts · Cashews · Peanut butter · Peanuts · Pecans · Tahini · Walnuts
ANIMAL PROTEIN	Beef · Carp · Clams · Fish · Lamb · Lobster · Mussels · Oysters · Pork · Rabbit · Salmon · Scallops · Shrimp · Tuna · Turkey · Venison
PASTA (WHITE)	Macaroni · Noodles · Spaghetti
BEANS AND LEGUMES	Black beans · Chickpeas · Green peas · Kidney beans · Lentils · Lima beans · Pinto beans · Red beans · Soybeans · White beans
OTHER	Alcoholic beverages · Distilled vinegar · Potatoes · Wheat germ

BETTER THAN SCIENCE FICTION

The powers that heal us are far more powerful than the powers that age and break us. Every single minute of every single day, 365 days a year, our bodies are adjusting and creating the necessary checks and balances so that our chemistry remains as perfect as possible. When our pH drifts lower than 7.35, we need to recognize that we are starting down a road of disease and poor health.

What kind of diet will allow the food we eat to naturally and successfully balance our chemistry? Since waste is a natural by-product of metabolism in every person, and since much of that waste goes unnoticed as it is eliminated, eating properly should keep our immune systems from being overstressed. We want our immune system ready to perform important work, not just cleaning up the garbage. It should be on alert, powerful, and ready to pick a fight with outside invaders, doing its assigned job. It shouldn't have to be reacting to continual internal battles that have been caused by unnatural conditions it was not designed to handle over the long haul.

Our immune system is so incredibly versatile that sometimes it seems more like science fiction than reality. Our immune system consists of lymphocytes, the white blood cells, which belong to two categories: B cells and T cells. Both of these types of white blood cells are like janitors. They clean up the debris that occurs from the natural metabolism of food. They get rid of dead cells and process metabolic garbage, rendering it harmless. They ingest harmful bacteria and rid our bodies of harmful viruses. Our eliminative organs (skin, lungs, kidneys, colon, and mucous membranes) continually send the waste and toxins out of our bodies.

A healthy body requires T cells and B cells to stand ready, much as a military reserve unit stands ready to defend and protect. They need to be ready, willing, and able to pick the right fights. When we are eating poorly and have therefore relegated our bodies to emergency protocols, our immune systems are chronically fatigued.

Among other outcomes, this can give cancer cells an opportunistic advantage although the problem may go unnoticed for a while. A compromised immune system leaves the body susceptible to all kinds of ailments, infections, and disease. (And that is why patients are often given T cell transplants or bone marrow transplants after a round of chemotherapy or radiation treatment.)

How can we better support our amazing immune systems? When we choose and consume good, living foods that are high in antioxidants, high in nutrition, and high in octane, our bodies produce minimal amounts of waste and our immune system disposes of it efficiently, like good janitors. If we happen to be invaded by a harmful type of bacteria such as streptococcus, our immune system engulfs it; our white cells ingest it, break it down chemically, and render it harmless. Cells that are dying and are floating around in our bloodstream get neutralized and taken away by more white blood cells. This is what the immune system is designed to do. When we get a cut, the immune system immediately comes to the rescue and starts cleaning and sterilizing the area, ingesting the toxic debris that can form in an open wound. We need to do whatever we can to keep our immune systems healthy and our systems balanced.

PROPER pH REQUIRES PLENTY OF CALCIUM—AND SLEEP

Another problem in maintaining proper pH comes from a most unlikely place. According to the latest research, sleep deprivation and a poor diet are almost inseparable. Sleeplessness is one of the earliest symptoms of a poor diet, and sleeplessness contributes to poor eating habits.[1]

As it turns out, getting a full night's sleep every night is vital to the maintenance of strong bones. It is estimated that the largest percentage of the bone replacement process occurs during deep sleep cycles. Getting enough deep sleep requires at least six to eight hours of solid sleep. How many people get that much? How many sleep even four hours at a stretch, deeply and without interruption?

This fact has important implications for the use of calcium within our bodies. Compounding the risk factors, postmenopausal women, for hormonal reasons, metabolize and absorb calcium less efficiently than premenopausal women.[2]

What kinds of food offer us the best opportunity to meet our calcium nutritional requirements? By now you know the answer. The most benefit will be from raw foods because the enzymes are active and bonded directly to the calcium molecules. When mineral-rich foods are cooked, the digestive enzymes attached to calcium get destroyed, and the human body's ability to metabolize and absorb the calcium is greatly reduced.

Which raw foods contain the most calcium? All deep-green, leafy greens and many of the juices, such as carrot and beet juice, contain high levels of calcium. Raw seeds and nuts, especially almonds, contain high levels of calcium.

What about supplements? Although we have become accustomed to the advice that vitamins and supplements are beneficial, they can become a crutch that people lean on while continuing to destroy their physiology with poor food choices. No amount of nutrition obtained in pill form can offset or correct toxicity, deficiency, or the effects of poor nutrition.

All cultures suffer from imbalances in their diets, although we would like to believe that some cultures' diets are superior to others. The French may have certain advantages over Americans, who may have advantages over Australians, who have advantages over Africans. The advantages must be defined in terms of which kinds of foods give us the "octane" the human body can burn the most efficiently without producing too much waste.

Milk, although at one time it was probably the most powerful food people could consume, loaded as it is with calcium to keep our bones strong and to stimulate proper organ function, has fallen from the "superior food" pedestal with the advent of enzyme-eliminating pasteurization. When you consider that the most industrialized countries of the world, in spite of very high consumption of dairy products, also have the highest bone-fracture rates and the highest osteoporosis rates, you have to wonder what's wrong with the picture. Meanwhile, the people in much of Asia and Africa consume little or no milk after weaning, very few dairy foods, and little or no calcium supplements. Interestingly, their fracture rates are 50 percent to 70 percent less than those of the Western world, and their osteoporosis rates are also significantly lower.[3]

A worldwide study correlated the number of hip fractures with the average amount of animal and vegetable protein consumed in various countries. Not surprisingly, as animal food consumption increased, so did hip fractures.[4]

Our bones need more than simple calcium supplements. Amy Lanou, PhD, assistant professor of health and wellness at the University of North Carolina, tallied the results of over a thousand research studies on dietary risk factors for osteoporosis. She concluded that the calcium-supplementation theory is "bankrupt" and that a better solution is to eat a diet of low-acid-forming foods, which will strengthen bones much more effectively.[5]

Since 1975, 136 clinical trials have documented the effects of taking calcium supplements as it related to osteoporotic risk factors. Approximately 66 percent of these studies showed that high calcium and vitamin D intake (as found in supplements), even if taken from childhood through adulthood, yielded no reduction in the number of fractures. In one study at Harvard, researchers surveyed diet and hip fractures among 72,337 older women for an eighteen-year time period. Their conclusion was that neither the consumption of milk nor high calcium supplements reduced fracture risk.[6]

RISKS OF ANIMAL PROTEIN

As strange as it may sound, your good bone health begins in the blood. When high-protein meat diets acidify your blood, your pH gets unbalanced. To counteract the acidic blood, your body must neutralize this acid to avoid serious problems, including osteoporosis. But to neutralize it, your body must draw from its own reserve of alkaline material, which happens to include the calcium compound that is stored in your own bones. This breakdown of your own bones forms that essential alkaline ash that balances the acidity. The calcium released from your bones eventually gets excreted in your urine.

If you rely on meat and dairy to supply your protein, the amount of acid that is created will add to the acid from the proliferation of microforms, causing in some highly prone individuals, mostly women, a depletion of calcium from bones that is faster than the new production of new bone matter.

The enormous concern about protein in the American diet has rendered us all but paranoid when it comes to getting our daily requirements met. Many people believe that you cannot get adequate protein if you don't eat meat. That is just not true. Although plant foods do contain enough protein to keep you healthy, you need to be taught what to consume on a daily basis so that in a week's time you receive complete protein.

Don't fool yourself into believing you have enough willpower to change your eating habits simply because you are motivated by vanity. Long-term change consists of permanent changes in your basic instincts, and even a desire for better health may not provide enough sustained motivation to achieve it. This makes self-preservation possibly the best motivator of all.

CHAPTER 12

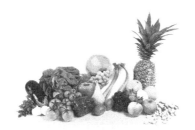

EXCITOTOXINS

Excitotoxins are neurological toxins, poisons that overstimulate neurons, and they enter our bodies through the foods we eat. Some of the latest findings have shown that excitotoxins are one of the leading contributors to neurological disorders such as Parkinson's disease. Neurons in our brain contain the transmitters and receivers that conduct instructions for locomotion as well as other higher levels of autonomic function, and this poison is directed against the vitality and health of neurons. The term *excitotoxin* sounds ominous, and for good reason.

If an excitotoxin is present in food, we don't experience any *apparent* negative effects. The word *apparent* is the key. We don't suffer any instantaneous or radical reaction to that ingested poison. We tend to look at our food in a very one-dimensional way; if it tastes good and passes uneventfully through and out of our systems, everything is OK. We rarely attribute disorders or maladies to something that tastes so good. Insidiously, without our awareness, excitotoxins can be disturbing the fine balance in our brain where bodily functions are regulated. Some of the latest studies are linking excitotoxins with chronic migraines.

MSG AND ASPARTAME

I'm sure you've heard of MSG (monosodium glutamate). It has been used for decades as a flavor enhancer. As it turns out, MSG is an excitotoxin. It is used to boost the taste of foods that would not normally taste good and to make even good-tasting foods taste even better.

Why do packaged foods taste better than foods naturally created out of the earth? A cucumber or a piece of celery or a carrot may fulfill your nutritional needs, but it might not satisfy your taste buds. The enjoyment we receive from the taste of processed foods greatly exceeds the satisfaction derived from the taste of plant-based natural foods. Glutamates enhance the taste and characteristic of foods, making them scream louder than their natural counterparts. When our taste buds come into contact with these additives, we develop a love affair with these tastes.

In the latter part of the twentieth century and the early part of the twenty-first century manufacturers have continued to use MSG in many types of processed food to improve its texture, taste, and ability to dissolve and create a pleasing sensation in our mouths. Foods that have been enhanced with MSG initially make our brains very happy. Our taste buds incorporate receptors called glutamate receptors, which allow our brains to recognize the ingestion of foods, such as mushrooms and tomatoes, which contain naturally occurring glutamates.

In a similar way foods that have been sweetened with aspartame (marketed under the name NutraSweet but also added as an ingredient to many processed foods) affect neurological health negatively. How does this work?

The brain orders the production and the distribution of hormones to regulate metabolism, the absorption and distribution of calcium, and the metabolism of glucose in the brain. A neuron is a cell that transmits and receives commands to initiate functions successfully and smoothly. Neuron pathways are vital to all of our somatic functions and some of our autonomic functions. But when artificially synthesized glutamates enter the system, these neurons become affected negatively.

In his book *Excitotoxins: The Taste That Kills*, Dr. Russell Blaylock shows that the introduction of artificially synthesized glutamates begins to cause neurons to atrophy, destroying their vitality and health and interfering with the highly calibrated function of processing and utilizing calcium and glucose, which stimulate the proper production and distribution of hormones.[1]

Our taste buds can't detect the difference. When we taste sweetness, for instance, in the form of processed sugar or artificial sugar such as aspartame, the receptors on our tongues send a signal to the brain: "It is like glucose." This appears to be a friendly substance. Thus, processed or artificial sugar passes the taste test and fools the brain.

WHAT ARE EXCITOTOXINS?

Amino acids serve as neurotransmitters in the brain. The human nervous system needs amino acid neurotransmitters to operate. But excitotoxins are amino acids too. As such they can cross the blood-brain barrier and excite the neurons of brain cells to a point of exhaustion and eventual cell death.

Over time, as one consumes MSG, aspartame, or another excitotoxin, a formaldehyde by-product from metabolizing these toxic ingredients binds with cellular DNA and causes DNA damage. It tends to stick to the DNA, and over time the formaldehyde accumulation causes massive cell damage, which opens the door to diseases of all sorts, including cancer.

Glutamate receptors or channels can be found within the brain and throughout the nervous system, heart, and intestinal tract. So it is not only the brain that is affected by excitotoxins over time. Eating a large quantity of MSG or drinking aspartame-laced liquid (such as diet soda) can result in an immediate negative physical reaction.

When you read a food label, you will rarely see the term "MSG." Instead you will find many other terms, such as "hydrolyzed vegetable protein," "hydrolyzed soy protein," "glutamic acid," "natural flavor," "textured protein," "textured vegetable protein (TVP)," "artificial flavor," "spice," "calcium caseinate," "sodium caseinate," "yeast extract," "autolyzed yeast," "yeast extract," and more.

You will need to look closely to find aspartame listed among the ingredient names on processed foods, most of them reduced-calorie beverages and foods such as diet drinks, flavored coffee and pancake syrups, instant hot cocoa mixes, and reduced calorie sweets. You must realize that aspartame is also used to heighten sweetness in safe-seeming products such as breath mints, chewable vitamin supplements, flavored water products, flavored iced tea mixes, breakfast cereals, meal replacement shakes, nutritional bars, and low-fat/low-sugar yogurt.

It is possible to purchase processed foods without glutamates, but don't be fooled if the ingredient doesn't appear at all, because manufacturers are not required to use the word *glutamate* if the additive is not 100 percent pure in its synthesized form. Unfortunately this leaves us at a disadvantage. We are forced to further our own education in areas that are difficult to navigate without a degree in chemistry.

Being aware of ingredients is not a foolproof guarantee for identifying approved ingredients. We recently had such an experience with a product we had approved and used for years. We noticed that this brand of bouillon broth cube had undergone an ingredient change. The manufacturer had replaced a natural ingredient with a substance called "textured protein." Textured protein sounds as if it might be good. However, it causes the same neural damage as other glutamates. It was a good thing that we had remained diligent regarding what is on the label. Lesson learned: every now and then we need to check the labels of favorite products for ingredient changes.

NATURAL PROTECTION FROM EXCITOTOXIC REACTIONS

Magnesium can help impede glutamates from overloading glutamate receptors. The people who have a low magnesium count are the most prone to acute excitotoxicity, as evidenced by sudden, severe digestive distress, headache, or even heart attack. Magnesium is important for overall health; it is vital to at least three hundred biochemical functions within your body. So getting enough magnesium is a good idea in general.

If you buy magnesium supplements, make sure you get one that will dissolve in water, because this enables easier absorption into the blood. Natural magnesium can be found in green, leafy vegetables, and it is also available in whole grains and many beans and nuts.

Ginkgo biloba may provide protection against excitoxicity as well. People take ginkgo biloba supplements to help protect against Alzheimer's disease and to reduce "brain fog."

Omega-3 fatty acids (best obtained from fish oil) can block excitoxins while also repairing cellular damage. Small doses of selenium (also available in supplement form) provide protection from excitotoxin attack for glutamate receptors. Brazil nuts are considered a good natural source of selenium; two or three Brazil nuts a day is considered sufficient for optimum selenium intake. In addition, some experts recommend red clover (available as leaves for tea, tinctures, liquid extracts, and capsules).[2]

Zinc, another mineral, can also help obstruct the glutamate receptor channels from excessive excitotoxin absorption. Many people are zinc deficient. To see if you are one of them, you can take a zinc taste test that uses a solution of zinc sulfate. If, when you taste it, you get an immediate bad taste, that usually indicates that you have a sufficient zinc level in your body.

EXCITOTOXIN DETOX

The first step in any detoxification effort is eliminating the toxin. Once you have been practicing, to the best of your ability, aspartame and MSG abstinence, your body will start to detoxify itself. Aspartame is easiest to recognize and avoid, because it is the primary artificial sweetener in hundreds of diet sodas, sugar-free sports drinks, and processed foods billed as "reduced sugar" or "sugar free." Please don't confuse aspartame with stevia, which is a natural, safe, plant-based sugar substitute.

To augment and ensure detoxification, Dr. Blaylock recommends milk thistle to help the liver eliminate all toxins. He also incorporates curcumin into a glutamate-detox program. Curcumin is the essential ingredient of turmeric. It increases bile flow as well as boosting DNA repair enzymes. To aid the liver, he also recommends taurine, an amino acid that contains sulfur, as well as vitamins B_1, B_6, C, and E.[3]

Truth and consequences

The consequences of excitotoxins are showing up in the neurological health of Americans. Increasing numbers of Americans have hand tremors and aren't able to move or use their hands in intricate movements such as threading a needle, handing a drinking glass to another person, picking up a pen, or writing legibly. These problems are not only age-related; they are also related to the degradation and destruction of our neurons through poisoning with excitotoxins. These disabilities portend a final collapse when the neural fluid commands can no longer be processed.

Parkinson's disease or other neurological diseases and maladies may suddenly appear. Heavy metals and excitotoxins cause many of these disorders. Over time excitotoxins damage the finely tuned communication system within your brain, impeding its ability to conduct, give signals, adjust, and regulate every function of your body.

Excitotoxins also inhibit the production and distribution of the hormones that act as instigators, reminding your body of its functions ("It is time to stand up, sit down, go to sleep...").

Hormones tell the cells what, where, when, and how to function. Without the production and proper distribution of hormones, your body is poorly regulated, and you may suffer from difficulties such as depression, lack of concentration, or the inability to solve problems.

Your immune system has approximately ten years of emergency reserves. If you had to fight an infection for ten years, your immune system would eventually tire or collapse. Your brain is much more elaborate and so finely tuned to disturbances that it doesn't require much for it to manifest the effects of poor diet, especially a diet that contains excitotoxins.

Poor sleep is often the result of a poor diet. Your sleeping habits become disrupted, and the quality of your sleep gradually becomes less restful and restorative. It is during the sleep cycle that most of the restoration and rehabilitation take place at the neurological level.

Cease and desist

So what can we do when almost all processed and prepackaged foods contain such dangerous substances?

Stop! The first order of business is to get back to the point where you can establish a love affair with natural foods. The only way you can do that is to appreciate the taste of natural foods. You can't appreciate that taste in the standard American diet because you have both desensitized and insulated your taste buds.

Get rid of the toxins in your body while you replace them with the nutrition found in whole, natural foods. An appreciation of the wonderful taste of a plant-based diet will return as your senses are awakened to the subtleties of natural aromas, textures, and flavors. These are the wonderful characteristics of foods you were designed to eat.

"I like McDonalds because…" "I like Burger King because…" "I like KFC because…"

Everyone has a reason why they have a favorite fast food, but every reason falls into one category—taste. The fast-food giants have engineered our tastes into unnatural directions, and they are hoping to capture enough of a clientele who would rather eat their product than someone else's. But that engineered taste is poisonous! We must be able to distance ourselves from poisons, and we need to know that our love affair with taste satisfaction is nonnegotiable.

People frequently ask me, "If you don't eat meat and dairy, and if you don't eat processed foods, then what do you eat"? I suggest that you take a two-week period of time and take a good look at the main course you eat each night. In that main course, the center of the meal, you will most likely find meat. Note how this portion of your meal is prepared. Create a food log of the specific way any meat product is seasoned. Most often people duplicate their meals two to four times in a two-week period. Do you? What are your tastes dictating?

At Birchcreek none of our sixty meals in sixty days are duplicated. We offer a diet of whole foods, mostly raw, some cooked, and with recipes that anyone can follow. There are incredible amounts of food available in the natural world, and they will far exceed the narrow list of choices you have made in your everyday diet. You may think that you have sophisticated tastes, but how sophisticated are you when you eat such a narrow spectrum of food choices?

It is so much easier to funnel your choices into a narrow spectrum of foods (driven by taste) instead of learning to enjoy a diversified diet. Examine your choices. Anything you have purchased and put in your refrigerator or cupboard is probably there because you like it (if not *love* it). If you unexpectedly found it missing one day, you would think about it and crave it. You have institutionalized your eating habits, and over the door of your institution you have inscribed, "I crave what I eat."

You can recondition and redirect your cravings quickly by making a new habit of preparing and eating meals from whole-food sources. Remember the way your brain gets programmed: (1) You are *introduced* to a new taste. (2) If you like it, you *accommodate* new foods by planning to eat them again. (3) Repetition leads to what I call *"nesting."* (4) This nesting is the development of a habit. When a neural path is conformed into a habit, finally that habit causes a new craving. It can be said that cravings are in many ways akin to addictions. We should be so lucky as to crave wholesome food. It is possible, but it takes practice. Now that you understand the playing field, you can use your new knowledge with wisdom to make better choices.

Rehab 24/7

What does a lifetime of indulging in glutamates and other excitotoxins do to our brains? Can you recover from the damage? The neurons that have atrophied are not readily observable. Where is the damage?

The good news is that as we experience damage from consuming these additives, we are also experiencing rehabilitation. When the brain suffers a trauma, the body immediately begins to restore and to rehabilitate operational status. If, for example, you suffer brain damage in the part of your brain that orchestrates walking or speaking, you would begin a process of rehabilitation in order to restore and recover your abilities. The purpose of the repetition of rehabilitation is to set down new pathways in nearby areas of the brain to take up the lost ability to perform the tasks. Rehabilitation trains different neurons, ones not originally intended to perform those functions, to create a new circuit.

A similar process is going on every minute of every hour of every day for invisible neural damage, but there are limitations. Scientists describe this degrading of our motor operation due to glutamate neuron atrophy as a "detrimental cascading effect." My engineering background helps me understand this better by calling it the "angle of incidence," which describes the collapse of the integrity of a surface. When a surface reaches its threshold of being able to maintain its integrity, it fractures and breaks apart.

As the ocean waves beat against the shoreline, the integrity of the sand's configuration, overwhelmed by the pressure of the waves, collapses. This is like an avalanche, because several factors influence a failure in the integrity of the surface before that surface collapses. Picture in your mind this scene: After pouring beach sand to form a mound, the base of the surface, or footprint, is established. The footprint image remains visible for a while as you pour more sand over the mound to increase its height. As you continue pouring sand, it finally collapses. The collapse shortens the height of the mound but broadens the overall "footprint" of the mound.

In much the same way, glutamates create damage in our neurological health. As neurological pathways are collapsing, other pathways are in rehabilitation, creating new and complete circuits. The collapses continue to expand the mound over a period of years. Although unnoticed, the ongoing ingestion of glutamates in sugarless gums, sugar-free sodas, and processed foods instigates the inevitable and noticeable final collapse. The angle of incidence is a collapse that approaches the point of no return.

Glucose operates as an escort system. The survival of the brain is entirely dependent on this transporter system. If it should malfunction, the brain can become deficient of both energy and the supply of neurological impulses, ultimately causing permanent neurological defect. Aggravated by poison, a tipping point is reached, and function is impaired.

Neurological sickness is not the same as having knee pain or a continuous muscle ache or a backache. We develop physical ailments that are many times transient. We have some control over other types of recovery, but not so with neurological disorders or diseases. Such conditions are often signs that things will get worse if we do not seek specialized help. Often times the diagnosis comes when the problem is well advanced.

This is why we should be supremely concerned about what we ingest, because synthesized glutamates and a host of other engineered ingredients do enter our brains and cause damage.

One size does not fit all. Many factors come into play to determine how sensitive an individual may be to an excitotoxin. Our genetic strengths or weaknesses leave some of us more or less prone to disorders. Why take chances?

NATURAL TASTES FROM NATURAL FOODS

We need to become more appreciative of the natural flavor and textures of natural foods rather than processed foods, since almost without exception most processed or packaged foods contain glutamates in one form or another. We have to know what the names glutamate hides under in order to avoid them. Here is an excerpt from an article entitled "Protect Yourself From MSG and Aspartame Excitotoxicity":

> The first line of defense against the two most commonly used and pernicious food additives, MSG and aspartame, is avoidance. However, complete avoidance is not possible for everyone all the time. MSG, monosodium glutamate, has been disguised with several different names. Aspartame or its primary constituent, aspartic acid, along with disguised variations of MSG, have even shown up in food products or supplements sold in health food stores!
>
> Eating out, you're sure to be taking in some MSG. Even if the restaurant doesn't add MSG to the food it prepares, MSG or disguised variations are sure to be within the foods purchased by the restaurant. Soups, gravies, and all liquids with MSG or aspartame will ensure a more rapid overload of excitotoxins than other forms of tainted foods.[4]

Enhanced sugar, spices, and toxins from the standard American diet dull our taste. Is it any wonder that the longing for taste satisfaction far outweighs our hunger? After all, our threshold of taste satisfaction has been raised to such a point that we are unable to recognize the wonderful, delicate taste of natural food. Only when our taste is satisfied, not even when our stomachs are full (and certainly not when our nutritional need has been met), do we stop eating. We crave what we eat! Our stomachs keep expanding and weight increases along with the need for more calories to maintain our demanding condition.

No longer able to detect the taste subtleties of natural foods, we dismiss them as less satisfying and never find out how well they could have satisfied our true nutritional needs. We respond to triggers that excite our appetite: sight, smell, and sometimes sound. Even a passing thought can trigger a nutritionally starved appetite. We could have eaten just an hour ago and end up indulging again by eating more foods that are of the taste-satisfying variety, such as candy bars, chips and dip, and many other salty and sweet filler items— just the types of snacks that are the most heavily laden with dangerous additives.

Let's begin to create the habit of healthy eating. You will be able to find almost any kind of natural food at the average American supermarket, and other sources are almost as easy to locate. You could even grow some of your own food if you have the time and space. You can rely on the Birchcreek program to provide you with a myriad of excellent recipes. Practicing a new way of cooking with these recipes can be a fun and delicious habit-producing hobby. As you find meals you especially like, repeat them often, and create a lifestyle of healthy eating. I guarantee you that if you practice this new way of eating for as little as one month, you will be happy to find that these new foods will have already become a habitual acquired taste.

CHAPTER 13

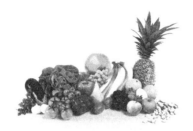

HEREDITY: IT'S MY PARENTS' FAULT

Whom do we blame when things go wrong? Is it all the fault of genetics and heredity?

Do you think that heredity is just a time bomb waiting to explode? Is it a matter of good or bad luck? Is it inevitable? What do you see when diagnosed with cancer or heart disease? Do you feel like a train in a tunnel with no way out, no wiggle room, waiting for nature to take its course?

In our twenty-first-century world no one needs to think this way. No longer is it about having enough courage to deal with what life might throw your way. Instead it is about knowing how to create a tipping point—heavily in your favor. As it turns out, heredity is not a hammer waiting to fall or a ticking time bomb; it is a tipping point!

When you see yourself in the mirror, you see your parents. Others may even tell you that you look like your mom or dad. You know you can't do much about your height, skin color, or prominent features. Along with most people you have come to accept the idea that you are doomed for whatever you have been genetically destined to endure. You may pat yourself on the back with some pride if you have a family that is relatively healthy. If you have slipped through the cracks of the defect factory and you think you are more complete, whole, or perfect than the next guy, you feel lucky. Although most of us have come from "factories" that are known for their high fidelity, we do need to pay attention to the care and maintenance side of health.

DIFFERENT MODELS AND MAKES, SAME PRINCIPLES

Take the automobile industry, for example. Ford, GM, BMW, and Mercedes manufacture products with particular strengths and weaknesses. When these cars come out of the showroom, they operate within the guidelines of the prescribed manufacturing standards, and by following care and maintenance guidelines, like the proper fuel and servicing intervals, these cars have a specific life expectancy. As long as purchasers operate them within the specific guidelines prescribed by the manufacturer, a 200,000- or a 500,000-mile warranty will protect them from expensive repairs. How a person operates that vehicle can alter and shorten its life.

Let's say we have cars of different makes, and they get

fueled from the same gas station—which has bad gasoline. Eventually the cars would begin to show effects in performance. At first, designated service visits would anticipate no serious ailments, but in time little things would begin going wrong. Maybe the Ford product might expel a little exhaust smoke. A GM vehicle might stall at the stoplight every now and then. When trying to accelerate, the BMW might have a little hesitation. A Mercedes may not demonstrate the same problems, because its manufacturing standards are so high and it can tolerate a little more. As troublesome conditions begin to manifest, the mechanic may change plugs, adjust timing, check wiring, clean injectors, and adjust fluid levels. Some of the maintenance is routine. Other vehicles might require repair, adjustment, or parts replacement. None of those quick fixes have identified the root problem; they have only adjusted for the symptoms.

The problem begins to compound itself. Initially, although high-octane gas may have been required, it was not used. That's very much how the human body deals with "low-octane" fuel. The higher the octane fuel, the higher the performance and the lower the emissions or waste.

You are as controlled by your genetic makeup as each make and model of car is controlled by its design and manufacturing process. The propensity for disease and malfunction can be more prevalent in one family tree than another, just as a car coming out of factory may be better equipped to tolerate different conditions. Your family tree, over a period of time, has engaged in different lifestyles that have led to genetic damage. Thus, the quality of manufacturing that maintains your health, vitality, and normal operations was damaged long ago. Scientific reports say humans have been consuming the wrong fuel for thousands of years. The result is not an opinion but fact.

OUR CELLULAR FACTORIES

We tend to regard ourselves as monolithic creations. In fact, we are made up of 100 trillion cells, all individuals in their own right. Each cell is part of a greater whole with specific function and traits. Our bodies continuously give birth to new cells. Not only perfect cells but also damaged cells are propagated—not that a cell is not capable of correcting small defects. Opportunity dictates a cell's ability to revitalize and correct the tiny bit of damage it experiences during daily functioning, and the regeneration of each cell within the life cycle of the human body is finely tuned to the organ from which it is duplicated.

Most people are *not* born with disease or life-threatening conditions. The majority of us have bodies that function normally, regardless of how weak or sensitive or imperfect our cells are. And yet cells that are prone to defect are governed by a time bomb type of mechanism or by a gradual deterioration in cellular vitality. This creates a tipping point when the cell can no longer operate as it was designed to operate at birth.

A family tree with multiple instances of cancer or heart disease highlights the propensity for these problems. One family may have a lot of cancer of the prostate; another family may have histories of breast cancer. Another family's members may have diabetes. These represent weaknesses in physiology at the cellular level.

THE TIPPING POINT REVISITED

Science no longer holds the theory that the genetics of cancer are like a time bomb. Cancer is a disease of opportunism. This makes cancer more of a "tipping point" disease. This tipping point comes from a lifetime of deficiency and toxicity caused by the consumption of foods that produce harmful effects.

Take obesity, for example. A terminally ill cancer patient will be thin and emaciated, but more patients started out obese or overweight in the early stages. Recent studies have shown definite risks in the correlation between obesity and cancer, as follows:[1]

- Kidney cancer in both men and women (two-fold increased relative risk)

- Endometrial cancer (one-and-a-half-fold relative risk)

- Postmenopausal breast cancer (twofold relative risk)

- Colorectal cancer (may be related to the low physical activity of obesity)

- Esophageal cancer (probably related to the gastric reflux of obesity)

According to one report, obese individuals have a 20 percent greater risk of developing colorectal cancer over those with normal weight. Obese men are at 30 percent greater risk of developing colorectal cancer compared with obese women. An Australian study showed that carrying even a few excess pounds or kilos greatly increases the risk of colorectal cancer;

for every five kilograms of weight gain, the risk of developing the cancer increased by 7 percent.[2]

Interestingly, obesity can be somewhat protective for two cancers: breast cancer in premenopausal women and lung cancer. Yet most studies of obesity and breast cancer survival suggest that obese women have poorer survival rates than women with less body fat. Being overweight or obese increases substantially the risk of dying from cancer, according to reports of the American Cancer Society.[3]

Overall, while the mechanisms underlying the obesity-carcinogenesis relationship are not fully understood, sufficient evidence exists to support recommendations that adults and children maintain reasonable weight for height and age. Prevention is always better than cure.

THE ROSETTA STONE

Medical science always seems to be on the threshold of great discoveries. But with any new advance it takes time to sort out truth from theory or myth. Early on, for example, it seemed logical to say that a high incidence of familial breast cancer indicated a predictable, inevitable genetic time bomb for female family members.

For an eight- to ten-year period after the BRCA (breast cancer) gene was discovered, tens of thousands of women in America voluntarily had mastectomies, hoping to avoid probable breast cancer. But not everyone with this gene defect develops cancer. Today this has become an obsolete solution, because it was only a preemptive measure against simply having the defective gene.

Now scientists have concluded that cancer and other

diseases occur as a result of deficiency and toxicity. Over time we have been diminishing the healthy viability of our genetic makeup. When the human body is put under stress and strain because of poor food choices, that tipping point, like a trigger, allows your weakest genetic link to break.

Here is an excerpt from a leading study on the subject:

> How do BRCA1 and BRCA2 gene mutations affect a person's risk of cancer?
>
> Not all gene changes, or mutations, are deleterious (harmful). Some mutations may be beneficial, whereas others may have no obvious effect (neutral). Harmful mutations can increase a person's risk of developing a disease, such as cancer.
>
> A woman's lifetime risk of developing breast and/ or ovarian cancer is greatly increased if she inherits a harmful mutation in BRCA1 or BRCA2....
>
> The likelihood that a breast and/or ovarian cancer is associated with a harmful mutation in BRCA1 or BRCA2 is highest in families with a history of multiple cases of breast cancer, cases of both breast and ovarian cancer, one or more family members with two primary cancers (original tumors that develop at different sites in the body), or an Ashkenazi (Eastern European) Jewish background.... However, *not every* woman in such families carries a harmful BRCA1 or BRCA2 mutation, and *not every* cancer in such families is linked to a harmful mutation in one of these genes. Furthermore, *not every* woman who has a harmful BRCA1 or BRCA2 mutation will develop breast and/or ovarian cancer....

It is important to note, however, that most research related to BRCA1 and BRCA2 has been done on large families with many individuals affected by cancer.... Because family members share a proportion of their genes and, often, their environment, it is possible that the large number of cancer cases seen in these families may be due in part to other genetic or environmental factors. Therefore, risk estimates that are based on families with many affected members may not accurately reflect the levels of risk for the BRCA1 and BRCA2 mutation carriers in the general population.... Therefore, the percentages given above are estimates that may change as more data become available.[4]

I have found nothing in any medical information that leads me to believe this defective gene carries an inevitable death sentence. The reference to the probable occurrence rate was higher than most other genetic mutation indicators but was by no means 100 percent guaranteed. As in all medical studies, poor physical conditions due to injury, diet, or lifestyle often precipitate or accelerate anticipated dysfunction or disease.

In other words, you may have been born with a mutated gene, but you were not born with cancer. After reading all the evidence, I believe cancers develop during a lifetime of eating foods harmful to our bodies. We have finite abilities to restore, repair, and correct function. Eventually we begin to lose the battle and yield to the less than perfect genetic condition found in the weakest link. Disease develops after a lifetime of cellular assault with pollutants, poisons, and deficiencies.

The DNA of each cell is susceptible to damage. Carcinogens are the most lethal poisons to enter cells. Continued cell vitality is essential in order to propagate healthy cell division and, thereby, healthy bodies.

DNA

DNA is biological language. It instructs, organizes, and conducts the operation of life. DNA, found in every cell, provides all the information necessary for a living organism to grow and function. The instructions come in the form of a molecule within each cell that is called DNA.

The structure of DNA is represented by a ladder twisted into a spiral shape (a double helix), with each rung of the ladder represented by a pair of bases. There are four bases—adenine (A), which pairs with thymine (T) and cytosine (C), which joins with guanine (G). You can think of each base as representing a letter, with the letters grouped in threes to form words and a number of words making a sentence, or a gene.

Although the bases are always in fixed pairs, the pairs can come in any order. This way, DNA writes "codes" out of the "letters" (the bases). These codes contain the message that tells the cell what to do.

DNA replication occurs when an enzyme called DNA helicase splits the DNA down the middle by breaking the hydrogen bonds between the pairs. (The "legs" of the double-helix ladder get separated into two single strands.) Then new strands are formed when another molecule called DNA polymerase matches each of the strands, pairing A with T and G with C, so that each copy of the DNA molecule is composed of half of the original molecule and half of new bases.

DNA is what tells the cell how to make particular proteins. Proteins do most of the work in cells and in the whole organism. Proteins are made out of smaller molecules called amino acids. To make a protein to do a particular job, the correct amino acids have to be joined in the correct order. A piece of DNA that contains instructions to make a protein is called a gene.

Mutations

When DNA is copied, mistakes sometimes occur, and these are called mutations. We find three main types of mutations:

- *Deletion,* when one or more bases are left out
- *Insertion,* when one or more extra bases get put in
- *Substitution,* where one or more bases are substituted for another base in the sequence

Mutations are not always bad for the organism. Sometimes they can be neutral, or of benefit. Sometimes mutations are fatal for the organism. If, for instance, the protein made by the new DNA does not work at all, this can cause an embryo to die.

Just imagine

Consider the size of a human cell, and consider the fact that a human being has about one hundred trillion of these cells. Then consider the fact that within these cells there is a microscopic strand of DNA that is infinitely smaller than the cell itself; imagine the amount of information that is on this biological encyclopedia of data. It is mind-boggling. If you were to unravel a single strand of DNA without damaging it, which you could not do, the length of that strand of DNA would be approximately six feet long! The density of information on this strand of DNA is almost inconceivable to the human mind. If we were to stretch out each strand of DNA contained in each of the one hundred trillion cells and connected them end to end, we could travel to our sun, ninety-three million miles away, and back six hundred times!

The amazing thing about DNA is that the DNA in my skin cell is identical to the DNA in the cells in my liver or my kidney or my lungs. Within the library of DNA there are instructions for a cell to function in a certain way when conceived in that organ or body part. DNA carries the identification, characteristics, and functions that match its location—skin, eye, liver, sinuses, and every other cell in the body. When a cell divides, the DNA replicates itself, thus maintaining the fidelity of the cell and of the organ, enabling it to function properly within a specific environment.

In other words, these cells have an identity, a timing, and a cadence. Each cell has a certain life expectancy and a certain rate of self-renewal. Skin is a rapidly recovering system of new cells, with new skin being created all the time. Mucous membranes are the same. But bones are very slow to recover. Still, over a one-year period much of a person's body is renewed. Over a seven- to ten-year period almost all of a body is renewed, except for brain cells and the cells of the nervous system in the spinal column. This incredible mechanism exhibits such consistency of performance that we are only beginning to understand its complexity.

READY...AIM...DON'T FIRE!

People have been made with slight differences, differing strengths and weaknesses, and different propensities for disease. If my family has a particular proclivity toward diabetes, my chance of acquiring diabetes is greater than the person whose family tree doesn't have any incidences of diabetes. Lifestyle choices (that our families pass on from generation to generation) increase our chances of resisting or acquiring maladies. As a consequence we may be genetically prone to disease, only to assist the disease process by what we eat. A diet leading to obesity and causing heart disease, cancer, and type 2 diabetes often follows a contiguous family line. Just as with a chain-link fence with weak links in it, a strain on the weakest link will cause it to break.

Toxic diets cannot help create a favorable cellular environment. The chances of avoiding diseases are naturally far better when people are eating the proper diet. In essence, eating the proper diet takes your finger off of the trigger.

If you are genetically prone to a particular disease or weakness in your physical makeup, you are positioned in the crosshairs of risk. But the "gun" does not have to fire. The trigger finger will be controlled by food and quality of life choices. Poor and unhealthy diets create a tipping point, and that dangerous tipping point occurs when that little added deficiency or toxicity makes your weakest link break down.

Eliminating meat, dairy, and processed foods from your diet is like taking your finger off the trigger! When you eat a plant-based diet, you have a better opportunity to overcome disease.

We have a tendency to consider ourselves sick only after laboratory tests return with abnormal results. A disease like type 2 diabetes almost always begins with insulin resistance. This condition goes largely unnoticed until it progresses to an elevated blood sugar. We were sick before we identified the full-blown disorder. But we do have warnings, the precursors to disease.

LETHARGY

People who attend Birchcreek often say they aren't exercising because their lifestyle doesn't offer enough time or they are just too busy. Or they say that they have too many hobbies, and exercise isn't one of them.

The truth is that they don't exercise because they have no energy. Our energy represents our cellular factory working at top efficiency, and the type of food we eat determines the efficiency of that factory. A highly efficient cell can produce energy with a minimal amount of waste. When we feel lethargic, it is because every cell in our bodies is suffering a drain of energy for that particular day, month, or year. Most of the time this lethargic condition is caused by a diet that is low in "octane."

From a genetic point of view, what is the consequence of eating a diet low in octane? The efficiency of the food you eat and the burning of that fuel for the production of energy directly affect the chemistry in your body. Nutrition must be fully burned and fully utilized with a minimal amount of waste. Then you feel like you have vitality with a storehouse of energy waiting and ready to be spent!

Lethargic people take whole days off from life sometimes. They don't have a pain or a particular malady; they just don't have the energy to perform normal activities. Whatever energy they do have gets applied to the simplest of tasks. Conserving energy becomes a priority. People who could walk prefer those automated carts seen at many stores. In a process of using the amount of energy it takes to walk for five minutes, their major muscle groups (starved of vital oxygen by their inactivity) make their legs "give out." Poor diet combined with inactivity results in obesity and places damaging pressure on joints, ligaments, tendons, and muscles.

Exercise is really needed. Once energy has been lost, strength diminishes, and then the ability to do basic things vanishes. If you have a loved one in this condition, love too often turns to labor, as he or she relies on your limbs to do what his or hers cannot. A prolonged decline takes its toll on a relationship that was once built on love and respect. Quality time turns into an all-day and sometimes an all-night job. Personal hygiene gets compromised as independence evaporates and loved ones must assume the total care of their family member.

What is not visible on the exterior is that lethargy happens on the genetic level. Each cell is a world within itself. As a poor diet and lifestyle slowly starve and pollute the environment in which each cell draws sustenance, each cell is affected equally, and they lose their ability to propagate with fidelity and vitality.

A skin cell that divides normally acts to replenish the skin. The new cell acts just like a skin cell. A new kidney cell does the work of a kidney cell. Every cell of every muscle acts like a muscle cell. This identity gives each cell specific work to do. Cancerous cells, however, have lost their identity and have become renegades, like a skin cell growing on an eye or a toenail cell growing in a lung.

Besides having a specific assignment, every normal cell has a specific time, a cadence in which it multiplies. But the timing of a cancer cell gets lost, and it multiplies more quickly than other cells do.

SAD BUT TRUE

A woman goes for her annual gynecological visit, and after an examination she is given a clean bill of health. Without symptoms or warning, the good news turns to bad at the next visit. She wonders what happened and why nothing was discovered previously. Last time it didn't exist. Last time she wasn't identifiably sick.

What has happened? Every cell in her body has strengths and weaknesses identified through its DNA. When those weaknesses are influenced by poor chemistry, cells lose their vitality. The enzymes within each cell that prepare the nutrition for the nucleus, the *organelles* that maintain the efficiency and repair of the cell, and the sentinels associated with each cell that identify damage and initiate repair—all of these capabilities comprise the chemistry of the cell. When this chemistry is polluted, a cell becomes lethargic.

As a result the body's ability to metabolize food becomes increasingly more difficult. The immune system gets extremely tired cleaning this polluted environment. Debris begins to build up, leaving little to help the cell thrive. The cell's life is threatened.

The cytoplasm, the fluid within the cell, must remain in a chemical condition that offers vitality to the cell. The squalor around it hardly fosters health and vitality. As long as the body was functioning properly because of a good chemistry, the cell was not under duress. Daily variations in chemistry cause great fluctuations in cell vitality. As eating habits change, so does the cell's vitality. If a person's genetic weakness falls in a particular category called cancer, then the cancer trigger ends up being reached as the cells' ability to maintain and regulate their smooth and efficient operation becomes compromised. After losing efficiency day after day, the cells reach the breaking point, the point at which they can no longer function the way they were designed to do. You may go for a medical exam and have specimens sent to the lab. You get a phone call with troubling results.

Cells that are no longer considered healthy can be identified as *cells in transition* or cells that are *precancerous*. These days early detection means we can peer inside a cell and recognize any changes taking place that could signal imminent danger. From a pathological point of view, we see the earmarks of cancer. We know what parts of the body are composed of fast-reproducing cells. The cells of the uterine wall, for instance, grow and get shed on a monthly basis.

In a petri dish, both cancer cells and bacteria thrive in a chemistry that is notoriously low in oxygen, with a higher-than-optimum degree of acidity. People who are in midlife or past it are in the time in life where cancer, a disease of opportunism, begins its waltz to prominence. Their body's defense systems are out to lunch, feeding on so much debris and pollution that they can no longer prevent and fight disease.

In the petri dish, when the low-oxygen, acidic environment is exchanged for a healthier oxygenated pH-balanced environment, we see a slowing or halt in the regeneration of cancer cells. Likewise, healthier cells thrive from the moment that chemistry is improved. Our immune systems thrive in a proper pH environment. This should lead one to a common sense assertion: foods that produce acidity should be avoided while foods that promote and offer high alkalinity should be copiously consumed.

Many symptoms go unnoticed. Even precancerous cells oftentimes show no evidence of deviant behavior. So it is not that cells aren't operating properly; they are just beginning to falter. When we begin to see visible signs or have physical symptoms, we may go to a doctor to find a cause. But the flip side to the ability of medical expertise is that often doctors are catching things that could have been prevented in the first place. I like science, and I appreciate medicine. However, I am frustrated with the continually increasing numbers of cancer diagnoses.

WHAT IF?

Early detection is important, but the mortality rate for cancer has shown little improvement.[5] Lives may be lengthened, but the majority of cancer diagnoses offer virtual death sentences. Consequently patients undergo earlier treatment for longer periods of time with the same result—premature death. To a dying cancer patient, it is hardly an improvement in the economy of the quality of his life when harmful poisonous chemicals and radiation leave him with several years of suffering and then death. Is this a fair compensation—to know early on that you have cancer (long before your mom or dad could have ever known)? Is it fair when you spend your life's earnings (and many times that of your family) in order to fight back? It is little consolation in the last stages of cancer to ask, "What if…?" "What if I hadn't relied on chemotherapy or radiation? What if I had just cleaned up my diet?"

CHAPTER 14

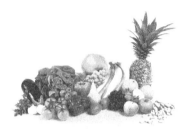

BEHAVIOR MODIFICATION

Let's engage in a little time travel. You're going to travel back in time to about 1850, and you're going to transport with you a lunch of processed, packaged foods. When you arrive, you meet someone and ask him to share your lunch. The two of you sit down together overlooking a pond situated behind a farmhouse. When you open your lunch box, packed with twenty-first-century food, your startled 1850 lunch guest sees your "food" and doesn't know what to do with it. To him it doesn't look or smell like food. In fact, to him it isn't food at all. He takes a few nibbles to be polite, but he instinctively knows better than to eat very much of it. We can predict that if he did—and he would be eating this kind of food for the first time—he would get quite ill.

Is your 1850s lunch guest merely a food snob, or is your old-fashioned friend much healthier than you, the time traveler? Should he modernize his diet? If he does, we can guarantee that he will become a toxic, overweight, cancerous, arthritic, hypertensive, diabetic, allergic, dysfunctional insomniac.

Our ancestors were closely tied to an agrarian lifestyle. Even if your father worked in a factory, farms were all around, and he was more influenced by an agrarian lifestyle than an industrial lifestyle. In order to move forward, we need to go backward and begin to eat more like our forefathers ate. They didn't have convenience foods. Such convenience leads to a population that barely knows how to boil water.

TOOLS OF THE FUTURE

At Birchcreek we offer all of the tools to move your future back into the healthy past. The tools are modified versions of the same tools that got us into this mess. Besides recipes, work-shops, and personal support, we offer behavior modification.

We Americans have made a hobby of eating. It has gone far beyond eating for nutrition; food has become our hobby, a lucrative industry, and even a love affair. And our love affair with food is what got us into this mess. We need to find a way to build on this passion as we change it into something health-bringing.

You may need to buy some new cooking utensils, and you will definitely need some new recipes. Delve into the recipes that we can provide for you, and make yourself a plan for breakfast, lunch, and dinner, selecting the natural foods that you think will be enjoyable, starting only with foods you know you will enjoy. From there begin to do what you have done in the past. Acquire a taste for other foods. Build on your success. *Enjoy* your new freedoms even as you enjoy leaving your old compulsions behind.

Clients who leave Birchcreek are provided with six months' worth of recipes and desserts. They can keep experimenting with the meal plans and following their taste buds. If you sacrifice your taste, you will fail. Studies have shown that even when people have their bodies surgically altered to significantly reduce food intake, they have a high chance of not maintaining their initial weight loss; something like 70 percent regain all the weight they initially lost. We hope to spare you that failure.

Our springboard to success is juicing. The Birchcreek Jump-Start Your Life program recommends a juice fast, as I mentioned earlier in the book. This can seem like a radical step to some people. A juice "program" would better describe the true essence of the plan, since a "fast" seems to indicate sacrifice or deprivation. The program consists of seven days of fresh juices—fruits in the morning, a combination of fruits and vegetables at lunch, and vegetable(s) in the evening. Each day requires approximately 8 pounds of fresh, near-perfect fruits and vegetables per person, processed through a Champion Juicer (probably one of the finest juicers along with the Jack LaLanne Power Juicer). The juice contains bioflavonoids, essential fatty acids, proteins, calories, and complex carbohydrates, all from living uncooked foods whose enzymes are ready to unlock all the nutrition.

Juicing offers near-miraculous results. The detoxifying process brings our taste buds to life, and it satiates us nutritionally. After one or two days into a juicing program at

Birchcreek, most guests can't finish their 16-ounce dinner juice. By the end of the third day their energy begins to soar, and hunger is nonexistent. Energy and vitality overflow. This feeling comes from having an empty digestive tract and the beginnings of restoration for a healthy immune system. By the end of the week body chemistry is well on the way to restoration.

Best of all, this is not a temporary fix. This is for life. The best is yet to come!

People are amazed when we tell them that we are more concerned with their long-term health than with the ten, thirty, or more pounds they want to lose. They are further amazed when they find out that the promised rapid, healthy loss of weight comes simply as the by-product of healthy, proper eating.

Our clients lose an average of 9.2 pounds in the first week (independently documented). This makes them very happy, but in order to continue weight loss or maintain an ideal weight, they are going to have to implement new strategies and develop new habits, after taking a good look at their current dysfunctional habits, cravings, and compulsions.

HABITS, CRAVINGS, AND COMPULSIONS

In order to evaluate your own world of eating habits, you must become your own psychologist as well as patient. No one can force you to change, stop, or begin anything, so you will need to engage your own will and motivations.

You are in command! After all, you have been making food choices all your life. Even when mommy was trying to shove a spoonful of spinach into your mouth while you were sitting in your high chair, you were letting mommy know what you wanted to eat and what you didn't want to eat. Be reassured that your adult decisions will be less traumatic and less confrontational than the food wars between mommy and baby.

You can modify your old habits and taste preferences, even if they are very well established. You really can acquire new tastes. At first, bitter leafy greens may taste less than pleasant to you, but if you keep eating them, you will acquire a taste for them and even begin to enjoy them. (I now enjoy leafy greens more than all those other foods, which fall into the categories of sweet or salty.)

You don't have to start by acquiring new tastes, though. When you are serious about changing your food choices, feel free to start with only the foods that already taste good to you. Keep your taste buds happy. You don't have to eat foods you think are bland, tasteless, or nasty tasting. I'm not telling you to substitute a carrot for your ice cream.

A foolproof way of changing your dietary eating habits without any conflict involves using psychological tools on yourself. Play along with yourself, and you will succeed. Start by eating what you crave already. Find healthy foods that taste good to you—and make a practice of eating them. In this way you can allow your own physiology to take command of your natural reactions and conditioning. You may not have realized that you already know how to create your eating habits, cravings, and compulsions. How do you think you developed all those habits and cravings you live with now? It was simple. You practiced eating foods you thought tasted great, and you kept eating them until you were hooked!

Break old paradigms

The word *paradigm* and the phrase *frame of reference* are almost synonymous. In order to begin changing eating habits, you need to understand that your old frame of reference, the paradigm you have always held, is no longer true. I introduced this idea in an earlier chapter.

You will be glad to find that your stubborn mind-sets can be altered when you displace the old outdated information with better new information. Most of us don't know why we hold certain beliefs, because information has entered our lives in subtle ways, including the two- or three-second messages we hear on television and a host of subliminal messages that come to us every day.

By using your God-given intellect, you can change your beliefs and have faith for more change. Your intellect is one of your best tools, and you will be able to overcome any obstacle and endure any hardship if you have faith. According to the Bible, "Faith is the substance of things hoped for, the evidence of things not seen" (Hebrews 11:1). Can you believe in a slimmer, healthier you? You can if your faith is grounded in facts. To succeed, you will need both scientific facts and faith in your ability to change with God's help.

Learn how your physiology works. Begin to understand your habits and cravings, and you will build your confidence. This will make the changes in your diet become part of who you are. Permanent change doesn't require an all-or-nothing approach, but it does require a "taking ground" approach. You can only take ground as you begin to understand how you got here in the first place.

HABITS, CRAVINGS, AND COMPULSIONS CHART			
	HABITS	CRAVINGS	COMPULSIONS
BREAKFAST			
AM SNACK			
LUNCH			
SNACK			
DINNER			
PM SNACK			

HABITS

What is a habit? A habit is a well-worn neurological pathway of activity that you no longer have to think about; it just happens. A habit is a behavior, something you may not be aware you are doing, like biting your nails or blinking your eyes when you're anxious. All of us have powerful habits (hard to break) and casual habits.

To identify food habits, you need to identify the foods that you obviously like and consume regularly. Which foods do you eat at certain times? What foods do you repeatedly eat during the week? For instance, if you eat an egg every morning, or even if you eat only one egg per week, you should identify the egg as a habit food. If you write these down, a pattern will start to emerge. In fact, you may begin to notice that most of the foods you consume are habit foods.

Do you routinely have a snack between breakfast and lunch? That snack is a habit. Go down column titled "Habit" of your chart and begin to fill in foods that are "habit foods" first. Do not go to any other category until you have finished the "habit food" section in all the time frames.

Next to the morning category, write down two to five foods you eat regularly for breakfast. Then write down the two or three most common snacks you might choose between breakfast and lunch. (Remember to write down only those food snacks that you eat on a habitual basis.) If you come up with a generalized category, such as "chocolate" or "chips" rather than a particular snack ("a Snickers bar"), you may learn something about yourself; you have a craving rather than a habit food. There will be more information about this later.

To identify all of your lunch habit foods, begin with the foods you most frequently eat and end with those you eat the least. Don't be exhaustive. Write down the first three that come into mind, and add a couple more if you are certain the "habit" criterion applies to them.

Move on to the period between lunch and dinner, and write down two or three of your most common snack foods.

Dinner foods can be a little more complicated to identify. Do you fix your own food? Do you sit down to dinner, or do you eat on the fly? Do you sit down to dinner at someone's house, or do you go out to eat? These factors make this category broader than the previous ones. Habit foods usually are not surprise foods. They are planned foods. It can be a little more difficult to discern the repetitious patterns in a week of dining. Jot down five categories of food that you might eat during your typical dinner. Include your main courses, cooked vegetables, breads, and salads. If you eat "a salad" or "bread" three or four times a week, or every time you go to a restaurant, call that a habit food.

The goal is to find out what you're eating and why. You aren't concerned with the quality (good or bad), only with finding out your specific habit foods. Don't judge; just jot.

CRAVINGS

A craving is something you really, really like! Nobody craves something that is unpleasant to the taste or other senses. You don't crave something that offers pain or creates discomfort. You crave things that indulge your senses and create a wonderful, pleasant by-product—satisfaction. The intensity of desire increases as you repeat the indulgence. In fact, you will begin to notice a physiological anxiety when you have not satisfied a craving in a while, in the form of both physical and mental discomfort. You may think you crave particular foods. But what are you looking for when you select those foods? What is more intensely satisfying about them?

As you write down a food in the craving section, don't be surprised if it also appears in your habit section. Scan the foods that you have in your refrigerator or your cupboard. If you do the shopping in your household, you are probably buying food that you like more than you are buying food that someone else likes. You want to be able to open the refrigerator or cupboard and see your favorite food there. If it is not there, you will feel disappointed. You might even say that you "crave" what you don't have. And you might actually go somewhere to get it as soon as possible.

COMPULSIONS

As you fill out the section on compulsions, focus only on this topic. You may need to take a piece of paper to cover the other parts of the chart to keep yourself from straying into the other parts of the chart.

Compulsion foods fall into two categories. The first category is for foods you cannot stop eating once you've started. You are physically able to stop, but the psychological urge to have more is so strong that it surpasses the craving level. The second compulsion category describes your response: you know it is useless to resist, so when you see the food, you eat it. You don't try to avoid the particular type of food or use your willpower to put up any resistance to the temptation before you. Which foods are your compulsion foods? Write them down.

I know about compulsive eating. I am a former junk food eater; I loved fast foods. When I was a child, my parents used to take my brother and me to an amusement park called Adventure Land. To this day if I get a whiff of White Castle hamburgers, I am propelled back to Adventure Land, and my mouth and every pore in my body craves a White Castle hamburger. At the end of each weekly visit to the amusement park my parents took us across the road to White Castle. White Castle purposely wafted the aroma of their fast food across the road to the amusement park to draw in customers. This became more than a pleasant little habit for us; it became a full-blown craving and later a compulsion. Before we would leave our house to visit the amusement park, my brother and I were craving those little burgers.

Fast-forward fifty years, and would you believe that once when I was driving back to the old neighborhood, all of a sudden I was caught off guard by the sight of that White Castle architecture in the distance. Although I had not eaten

White Castle food in over twenty years, the mere sight of those towers created an instinctive reaction. I began to salivate.

Apparently, even today, driving the highways on Long Island, New York, and seeing out of the corner of my eye the distinctive White Castle façade, I am compelled to stop the car and have one. Why? It falls into the second compulsion description. My White Castle compulsion has already passed the threshold of habits and cravings, and it has become embedded deep inside. Having created a neurological pathway ever so long ago, any reminder of that taste triggers an instantaneous response. I could be in a rush or have an appointment, but I would reason that another six minutes would not matter—I would not miss the opportunity to enjoy that taste!

I have learned not to respond to that compulsion, having come to understand why and how my body operates and the reasons why I eat. I've learned how to avoid certain things and how to fortify against other things so that my compulsion will subside.

Alcoholics (people who crave alcohol) can go to AA for help, get sober, and recover. But to stay in recovery, they have to distance themselves from the social environment and the physical stimuli that would tempt them to fall back into old patterns. After going through withdrawal, a recovering alcoholic can't turn around and go to a bar with his buddies two weeks later. New habits and new cravings must replace the old ones.

It is no different for a person with food cravings. Part of distancing oneself from making poor choices in food (which are often compulsive choices) means building new habits and new cravings with healthier food.

Now that you have your chart completed, all of the foods in their categories, and are ready for change, you will begin to deconstruct old routines and begin building bridges to powerful and healthy replacements.

OUT OF THE DARK AND INTO THE LIGHT

Take a good look at what you have listed on your food chart. Are all of these foods junk foods, or are some of them actually good ones? Next to any food on your chart that you think is a good choice, draw a heart. Then place an *x* next to any food you think is a bad choice. At this point in your journey you should be able to accurately pick the healthy (good) food.

You see, those are foods you already love. They will become a key part of your strategy for successfully changing your eating habits. You do have the ability to make a change, and you will feel conviction if you do not follow through. You are no longer in the dark. In a way, you are without excuse.

Assume for a moment that I can take a person from this present reality in which we live and place him in a world where lung cancer, urinary tract cancer, and the bad effects of smoking don't exist. He has never read information about cancer or known anyone who died from cancer. He is a smoker.

When I tell him to quit smoking cigarettes, he says, "Why?" I seem to be ordering him to stop for no good reason, and I have offered no evidence to prove my point. In his mind smoking is nice; he likes the taste of it, it is a social habit, and it gives his hands something to hold.

However, if tell him that I think he should quit smoking cigarettes *and* I supply him with the scientific data about what smoking does to a person's body, he would then have a reason to contemplate a serious decision to stop smoking. *Truth* will give him a reason to change or begin the process of changing his frame of reference, his model of understanding, his paradigm about his smoking habit.

Asking people to change their diets is almost as difficult as the scenario just described. Lacking the ability to see beneath the surface of our habits and cravings, we don't see why we should stop eating certain foods. Look at a dessert that you may have put on your chart in any of the columns. Most likely it is taking up a lot of time and space in your diet and creating a lot of harm. If you like ice cream and are like most people, you have a special ice cream, and you like to eat it at a special time. If the craving hits you and you don't have it, you might even get in your car and go out and get it. If it is a compulsion, you are going to find the opportunity, and once you get it, you may finish the whole container. Ice cream holds a very special place in many people's "really like" department.

What can you do to wean yourself from your well-established pattern?

STRATEGIES THAT WORK

Breaking a habit is like tearing something out instead of unscrewing it. When you unscrew a bottle cap or a light bulb, you must do it carefully so that you can replace it later.

If you rip a bad habit out if your life, all you can do is throw it away. Lacking a suitable substitute, your resolve may weaken over time. Breaking a habit is a tearing, ripping action and then throwing the habit away. Even when we attempt to change our habits by exchanging one habit for another, we can meet with only marginal success if the new habit is less enjoyable to us.

For example, if you like to crochet, but your hands hurt so you're unable to hold the crochet hook, you might decide to substitute flower-arranging as a hobby, thereby maintaining a level of creativity in a less painful way. But what if you discover that you really miss the creative act of manipulating the soft yarn into something beautiful? Your substitution will be less than satisfying if the replacement activity isn't as enjoyable as the original.

A hint for habit breaking is *don't!* Not without carefully replacing the unwanted habit with something that appeals to the same senses.

Let's examine your habit of eating ice cream around eight o'clock every night (or every other night or just on Saturday nights). You have fallen into a habit of eating a large bowl of high-fat, high-sugar dessert. If you decided that ice cream is not good for you and that you are going to break the habit by having a fresh carrot instead, I think you can see that your strategy would not work. Even if you took the same bowl and filled it with a wonderful salad instead of the ice cream, it would fall far short of the comfort, satisfaction, and characteristics of your favorite ice cream. You are going to have to replace a dessert with another dessert.

At Birchcreek we devised an outstanding fruit sorbet dessert made from frozen mangos, bananas, and strawberries topped with carob honey syrup. Our guests have rated it as one of the best-tasting treats they have ever tested. By replacing ice cream with our recipe, you are keeping a routine that you enjoy—but replacing the food. Ice cream is dangerously high calorie, high fat, and addicting. Our sorbet is dairy free, fat free, healthy, and nonaddicting.

You see, it has to taste good, and it has to be in the same family. To change an ice cream habit, it has to be a dessert, preferably one of the same consistency. Our goal is not to simply break the bad habit but to change it into a good one. In a way we are not changing the habit, just the ingredients. By making substitutions such as this one, you can eat healthier foods, and you can even forget about calories. Even if you start out with a plant-based diet that consists of 60 percent raw and 40 percent cooked foods, and you can improve that to 75 percent raw and 25 percent cooked, you will lose weight, feel great, and have more energy to burn.

You may not need to make a substitution for every single food item. Another simple strategy for taking charge of your cravings and compulsions is to answer the question, "Which of the x foods can I consider never eating again?" You will find certain foods on your list about which you can simply say, "I won't really miss it." With your chart giving you insight into your own preferences, you will be surprised how quickly you can make changes in what you eat. Your own awareness of why you eat, when you eat, and what drives your appetite will empower you to make changes you never thought possible.

You are trying to create a personal strategy that is preemptive. You want to plot a different course, to avoid the familiar road, to create different avenues to get to where you are going. In order to distance yourself from the opportunity to be affected by something, it must be left behind in a significant way. With compulsions, which are not quite the same as habits or cravings, but rather foods of opportunism, you will need to avoid the opportunities in a strategic way.

To the uninformed, the ease of satisfying tastes and the convenience of grabbing food on the run makes eating poorly almost unavoidable. As more people are learning about healthier living, a new day is dawning.

CHAPTER 15

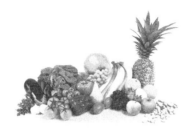

INTERCEPTING THE
TIPPING POINT

When most of our clients at Birchcreek come to us, they are relying on many prescription medications to assist with the functions their bodies are failing to perform normally as well as medications for comfort and pain relief. Some conditions are superficial, and some of them serious (cancer, heart disease, diabetes, osteoporosis, fibromyalgia, migraines, allergies, and many more). They come to Birchcreek expecting to lose weight, and they are surprised when their many symptoms begin to lessen, some to the point of complete elimination. They come to detoxify, and they find that their overall health improves by learning how to eat properly. Needless to say they are delighted with the results.

The number of people getting relief from their ailments and restored health and vitality is far superior to what any medical or fad diet can achieve. No prescription drug can claim the cures and the reversals that a good healthy diet and lifestyle provide. Often doctors call us to ask what we are doing and how we facilitate such an incredible change in their patients' well-being. At times we have flown across the country to meet with our clients' doctors. They want to know more about what happens here. How can people with a nonclinical medical background offer something that works better than anything science or medicine has to offer?

It is *not* because the food or juices we are serving are cancer cures or contain miracle powers. Rather, they are restorative agents. Your body is the miracle! The secret is its miraculous ability to repair itself, to regenerate, and to restore well-being. And yes, when we explore the nutritional and innate properties of a plant-based diet, we do find miracles locked within the food as well.

Sickness and disease are not inevitable, but they can be intercepted, avoiding further damage. We embrace the advances of early detection and interception with new and improved drugs, radiation, and surgery, but we also know that if you feed your body the kinds of food that it was designed for, you will both cleanse it and restore it to health and vitality.

CANCER-FIGHTING FOODS

Cancer is like the terrifying monster under the bed—and sometimes it becomes all too real. Specific natural foods can help in the fight against cancer. For example, certain foods carry unique properties; when eaten in sufficient quantities, they can become angiogenesis inhibitors. *Angiogenesis* means the development of new blood vessels, which is ordinarily a function of a healthy body as it heals wounds and keeps blood circulating to all organs and limbs. But when cancerous tumors develop, angiogenesis becomes a negative attribute as tumor growth is supported by a rapidly branching supply of new blood vessels. A cancer sufferer wants to employ anything that might interfere with the cancer's support system while also attacking the cancer directly. These plant and plant-based foods, if consumed in large quantities, can help.

ANTI-ANGIOGENIC FOODS[1]		
Green tea	Dark chocolate	Soybeans
Artichokes	Tomatoes	Strawberries
Blackberries	Raspberries	Blueberries
Cranberries	Garlic	Apples
Pineapple	Cherries	Oranges
Grapefruit	Lemons	Red grapes
Red wine	Kale	Broccoli
Cauliflower	Brussels sprouts	Bok choy
Ginseng	Licorice	Lavender
Turmeric	Maitake mushrooms	Ginger
Parsley	Pumpkin	Olive oil
Grape seed oil	Nutmeg	

This is just one example of a verifiable benefit from the consumption of a plant-based diet. If this good news were more widely known, not only the cure but also the prevention of serious, life-threatening diseases could become a reality. We do not give enough credit to the power of living foods combined with the healing power of our own bodies. Perhaps you and I will live to see the day when the medical community embraces the incomparable value of a plant-based diet. Wouldn't it be wonderful if our personal testimonies and efforts could bring that day sooner?

Change can occur. It has occurred in other areas. For instance, cigarette commercials in the middle of the twentieth century gave us the illusion that smoking was "cool." No longer is this the case. I'm eager to see the demise of the fast-food commercials of the twenty-first century. It is as if they are offering poison to children, and poisons become their favorite foods. Unfortunately fast food is so cheap that a mom can feed her entire family for so much less money and hassle than it takes to acquire, prepare, and feed her family with healthy foods. What's a mother to do?

CHANGE FOR THE BEST

At Birchcreek we try to give our clients the greatest measure of a jump start, allowing their own body's systems to restore, rebuild, and maintain life, keeping it vigorous and healthy into old age. Along with wholesome food, we provide wholesome knowledge.

Through initial detoxification we "reboot" people's physiology. We literally take down a person's operating system and remove its old programs. In as little as three months a person can be far along on his or her way to having a healthy, thriving life. When a person brings the operating system back up, new and improved programs get selected and installed, and once the person's system is up and running again, everything feels like new. We also teach them how regular detoxification will maintain an efficient operating system.

The choice of "new and improved programs" is all important. People must install uncorrupted "programs" of eating and living. Our healthy eating workshops are designed to take people step-by-step into a new way of eating, telling them why as well as how, so they can more easily embrace a new diet of highly nutritious plant-based foods.

Once a person's body "reboots," we encourage the person to install the equivalent of virus protection, which is knowledge, understanding, and the wisdom to implement their new dietary lifestyle. When you repair or buy a new computer, you are anxious to protect it from unwanted intruders. Virus protection either disallows imminent danger, or it alerts you to it. In the case of our bodies, we can be alerted through newly acquired and well-explained knowledge, which helps people grow in the wisdom necessary to implement good decisions.

We believe most people could do this alone, but many people do need support, and to get it, they need to stay connected. In a way Birchcreek's Stay on Track program, which I have mentioned throughout the book, is like an insurance policy for a person's investment in his newly rebooted operating system. With others walking alongside, he finds it much easier to take care of himself and to maintain his new lifestyle with enthusiasm.

CHAPTER 16

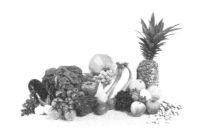

THE PROTEIN GAP

The word *protein* comes from the Greek word *prōteios*, which means "first" or "primary." Protein is indeed the primary ingredient of our well-being. Proteins make life possible. Proteins serve as enzymes, hormones, structural tissue, and transporters of various molecules.

Constructed like long chains, proteins are comprised of amino acids. Our bodies can manufacture some essential amino acids, but the rest must be supplied by the foods we eat. The amino acid components, even in the complete protein of animal foods, must be rearranged and reassembled for use by our bodies.

From the early twentieth century until after World War II, Americans were encouraged to eat more than one hundred grams of protein daily. As it turns out, nobody needs that much. Among the hazards of high-protein weight-loss diets, for example, are increased calcium stones in the urinary tract, kidney disease, some cancers, and, counterintuitive as it may seem, osteoporosis (because protein-rich diets cause people to eliminate more calcium than normal in their urine).

People are obsessed with worry about protein deficiency. Protein supplements, sold in health food stores as powders, drinks, or capsules, are very popular. While it is true that protein is one of the most essential nutrients we require to build and maintain function in our bodies, eating so much protein exceeds necessary thresholds.

GETTING ENOUGH COMPLETE PROTEIN

From a popular viewpoint, meat is the primary source of protein. However, a varied diet of beans, lentils, grains, and vegetables contains all of the essential amino acids. Up to recent times nutritional specialists thought that various plant foods needed to be eaten together in order to obtain their full protein value. Current research suggests this is not the case. Many nutrition authorities, including the American Dietetic Association, now believe that a person's protein needs can easily be met by consuming a wide variety of amino acid sources over a twenty-four-hour period. However, a person whose diet is not varied enough would do better to consume foods that contain the right combinations of amino acids at one time (like one-stop shopping) in an effort to obtain efficient protein.

For years it was believed that athletes need considerably more protein than the average person. In fact, athletes need only slightly more protein, and even from a vegetarian diet they can obtain plenty. Both athletes and nonathletes can get enough, but not too much, protein simply by replacing animal products with grains, vegetables, legumes (peas, beans, and lentils), and fruits, eating a variety of plant foods in sufficient quantity to maintain a normal body weight.

How much protein do you actually need? The federal recommended daily allowance tells us that for every pound of body weight, you need 0.36 grams of protein.[1]

How does this translate into real terms? A male between the ages of twenty-five and fifty who weighs 170 pounds would have an estimated caloric requirement of about 2,900 calories a day—61.2 grams of which should come from protein. (And remember, the older you are, the less protein you need.) So a young 170-pound male who needs 61.2 grams of protein per day would need to eat only 245 protein-derived calories per day. (You arrive at this number by multiplying 61.2 grams by 4 calories.) When divided into 2,900 calories, that number of food calories represents only 10 percent of the calories needed every day. In other words, we need only very small amounts of protein per calorie.

It is no surprise that the average vegan who does not understand what he is trying to do can take in less protein than the average meat eater. But by being informed, vegans and vegetarians can easily bring up their number of grams of protein into a better range.

Every whole food contains protein. Almost every vegetable and all plant-based foods contain a measure of protein, even carrots and celery. (A plant-based diet is so healthy because not only is it low in calories, but also 40 to 50 percent of the calories in it contain protein.)

Since cooking the food reduces the effectiveness and the amount of nutrition, you should eat your vegetables and fruits raw whenever possible. For example, 100 calories of cooked broccoli has about 6.8 grams of protein, while 100 calories of raw broccoli delivers about 11.2 grams of protein. (By contrast, 100 calories of beefsteak equals about 5.4 grams of protein.)

Where does protein come from?

Protein is derived from the action of sunlight on plants, which causes them to generate amino acids. Photosynthesis represents the only method on this planet that protein can be manufactured naturally. (The protein in animal foods has its origin in the plants that the animals ingested.)

Amino acids are assembled into proteins like multicolored beads on a string, with the colors representing the variety of amino acids needed to make a complete protein. Your body must reassemble a large number of amino acids to make up a complete protein. We are unable to use all the protein we eat because it has been cooked, damaged, and destroyed and cannot be reconstructed. If in the cooking process the amino acids have been damaged, the reconstruction of full, complete protein is stopped until we eat some foods containing more of the needed amino acids.

Meat is considered a complete protein, but is it efficient protein after it is cooked? Cooking renders some of the goodness in that meat unusable through destruction of amino acids. In any case, when a person takes in complete protein, the body disassembles it in order to reconstruct it for human use.

I am convinced that high-quality plant-based protein surpasses the value of the complete protein of meat, allowing for the steadiest synthesis of new proteins, and that it is therefore the healthiest type of protein.

Protein is a vital nutrient, no doubt about it. The body, while it stores quantities of fats and carbohydrates, cannot store large quantities of protein, so proteins must be consumed daily, as they are used up daily in an ongoing reconstruction process. However, protein cannot be used directly by the body until after it has been digested and broken down from its food source into singular amino acids, which then are recombined into usable protein.

For an excellent resource about meeting your protein needs with an all-plant-based diet, I recommend *The China Study* by T. Colin Campbell and Thomas M. Campbell II.[2]

CHAPTER 17

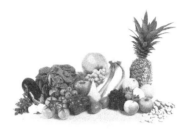

WORKING TOGETHER

I was looking through a local paper from an upstate New York town that represents a typical rural environment in America. I stumbled across the obituary page, and I happened to notice that the men on the list had died at forty-seven, sixty-nine, sixty-four, fifty-three, and sixty-one years of age. The women listed were eighty-nine, eighty-one, seventy-seven, and eighty-four when they died. It made me wonder again why women, on average, outlive men. I know that women tend to remain more active than men, especially in their senior years, and that women's bodies have not usually been physically injured as often as men's. In addition, men seem to be attracted to certain types of foods that are not good for them. They eat more than women, they drink more alcoholic beverages, and they express a preference for animal products, all while becoming more sedentary. As diet and activity go, so goes life expectancy.

By comparison, in nature all mammals live eight to ten times their maturation age. That means that you can figure their average life expectancy by multiplying their maturation age by eight or ten. (According to this measure, it could be said that we should live twice as long, depending on how you figure a human maturation age.) While medicine, science, and civilization have eliminated some of the diseases and the unsanitary conditions thrust on us, we can hardly imagine our lives without the diseases caused by our diet. What could our average life expectancy be if we avoided the foods that shorten our lives?

Many advocates of uncooked, plant-based diets cite an early study called the Pottenger Cat Study, in which Dr. Francis Pottenger demonstrated that when cats were fed cooked food diets, they suffered from congenital abnormalities, shorter life spans, and, within several generations, loss of reproductive capabilities.[1] In other lab experiments, mice that were fed a living food diet lived 50 percent longer than mice that had been fed cooked foods.[2]

GROWING CORROBORATION

I have come to appreciate both the pain and emotional stress people endure in overcoming their poor health and the joy of finally achieving their goals. In spite of the fact that I myself experienced the desperation and panic of not knowing what would become of me if I were to fail again at reversing my ill health, no one could have convinced me that eliminating meat, dairy, and processed foods would make such a positive difference. It was not until I came across some physicians who had blazed an unorthodox trail and put their professions on the line that I gave any credibility to a plant-based diet. In my opinion these men are the vanguards of twenty-first-century medicine:

Neal Barnard, MD

Dr. Barnard is the founder and president of the Physicians Committee for Responsible Medicine (http://www.pcrm.org). He is an author who examines clinical research studies and interprets the results nutritionally, and he is "an advocate for health, nutrition, and higher standards in research."[3] In his words, "If you change to a vegan diet, and do it vigorously, you have enormous power."[4] He believes that this is how people can prevent most cases of cancer and a host of other diseases.

Joel Fuhrman, MD

Dr. Fuhrman specializes in nutritional treatments for obesity and chronic diseases such as heart disease. He has authored many books, including *Fasting and Eating for Health: A Medical Doctor's Program for Conquering Disease* (1995); *Disease-Proof Your Child: Feeding Kids Right* (2006); and a two-book set, *Eat for Health: Lose Weight, Keep It Off, Look Younger, Live Longer* (2008) and *Eat to Live: The Amazing Nutrient-Rich Program for Fast and Sustained Weight Loss* (2011). Dr. Fuhrman, a former world-class figure skater, has appeared on many TV and radio shows.[5]

John McDougall, MD

Dr. McDougall is a physician and nutrition expert who has been teaching for more than thirty years the way to better health through a vegetarian diet. His books include *McDougall's*

Medicine: A Challenging Second Opinion (1988); *The McDougall Plan: 12 Days to Dynamic Health* (1991); *The McDougall Program for Maximum Weight Loss* (1995); *The New McDougall Cookbook* (1997); *The McDougall Program for Women* (1998); and *The McDougall Program for a Healthy Heart* (1998).[6]

Russell Blaylock, MD

Dr. Blaylock is a retired neurosurgeon best known for his opposition to MSG and aspartame. He has been a guest on numerous radio and television programs, and he is the author of many books and other publications, including *Excitotoxins: The Taste That Kills* (1994); *Health and Nutrition Secrets That Can Save Your Life* (2002); and *Natural Strategies for Cancer Patients* (2003).[7]

T. Colin Campbell, PhD

Dr. Campbell coauthored the book *The China Study* with Thomas M. Campbell II, a book based on decades of research. He is an emeritus professor of nutritional bio-chemistry at Cornell University and has established the T. Colin Campbell Foundation based in Ithaca, New York, to offer "the best scientific and health information available to the public, without influence from industry or commercial interests."[8]

Robert O. Young, PhD

Along with his wife, Shelley Redford Young, Dr. Young, a microbiologist and naturopath/nutritionist, is an author and public speaker on the subject of health, especially on the topic of pH balance. His books include *Back to the House of Health: Rejuvenating Recipes to Alkalize and Energize for Life!* (2000); *Sick and Tired?: Reclaim Your Inner Terrain* (2000);

The pH Miracle for Diabetes: The Revolutionary Diet Plan for Type 1 and Type 2 Diabetics (2005); *The pH Miracle for Weight Loss: Balance Your Body Chemistry, Achieve Your Ideal Weight* (2006); and *The pH Miracle: Balance Your Diet, Reclaim Your Health* (2010).[9]

Norman W. Walker, PhD

Dr. Walker (1866–1965) was a pioneering advocate of the use of raw juices for the sake of health. He established the Norwalk Laboratory of Nutritional Chemistry and Scientific Research in New York in 1910 and pursued a variety of other ventures during his long life. During his lifetime he published extensively, and after his death his books have continued to be revised and released, including the following: *The Natural Way to Vibrant Health* (1972); *Fresh Vegetable and Fruit Juices* (1978); *Colon Health: The Key to a Vibrant Life* (1979); *Pure and Simple Natural Weight Control* (1981); *Become Younger* (1986); *The Vegetarian Guide to Diet and Salad* (1995); and *Raw Vegetable Juices: What's Missing in Your Body* (2003).

Edward Howell, MD

The late Dr. Howell has been called the "father of food enzymes" because of his groundbreaking research, beginning in the 1930s and 1940s. He proved that food enzymes should be considered essential nutrients and that the heat of cooking can destroy them. His theories were published in two books that are still in print: *Enzyme Nutrition* (1985, revised 1995) and *Food Enzymes for Health and Longevity* (published posthumously in 1994). Dr. Howell advocated a diet of at least 75 percent raw food and supplemental digestive plant enzymes taken with the remaining cooked food to replenish what he referred to as the "enzyme bank."

All of these referenced materials have been part of the driving influence in the creation and philosophy of the Birchcreek Jump-Start Your Life program. We owe a debt of gratitude to the researchers and dedicated practitioners who have provided a foundation on which we can build. These doctors have motivated me to apply over three thousand hours of study to develop a program that delivers detoxification, nutrition, and strategies to change a person's life. These are the doctors who have documented and validated the science behind what I try to explain in everyday language through eight hours of classroom time and six hours of workshops. My goal is to teach in a way anyone can understand and retain the information.

Throughout the Birchcreek programs and throughout this book, I have relied heavily on the books above (and more) by these medical and nutritional professionals.

APPLYING THE FINDINGS

Standard weight-loss diets warn people not to lose more than 1 to 1.5 pounds per week for fear of nutritional depletion. But balanced, plant-based diets have historically outperformed those diets without risk of dehydration, deficiencies, or chemical imbalances.

If you are eating the standard American diet and wish to lose weight, rearranging the foods that you do eat to diminish caloric intake is only marginally effective. Merely reducing the volume of food in some way simply delivers less nutrition than you were getting from an already deficient diet. You need more nutrition, not less, when you are dieting. With careful attention to nutritional quality, rapid weight loss is safe. In the Birchcreek Jump-Start Your Life program, rapid weight loss is healthy because two major risk factors are being addressed: deficiency and toxicity. While clients get an abundance of nutrition, they also get a continuous, steady level of detoxifying.

No fat is added to the foods, so the only fat in the diet is what occurs naturally in the food. This diet has about 5 to 10 percent fat, zero saturated fats, 25 to 40 percent protein, and 50 to 70 percent carbohydrates. Food choices are very low in fat and high in fiber. Calorie-to-protein ratio is significantly improved over previous diet plans. Although you eat enough to feel full, your calories are very, very low and well spent, making nutrition and aggressive weight loss very compatible.

With the Birchcreek Jump-Start Your Life program, a person who is thirty to sixty pounds overweight can expect to lose nine to ten pounds the first week and about five pounds the second week. People who stay on this program until they get close to their ideal weight can continue to lose about a quarter of a pound a day. (Weight loss slows down as a person approaches ideal weight.) Starvation cannot produce this kind of results because the body will go into starvation mode for survival, slowing down bodily functions and reserving the fat stored in the body instead of burning it.

How do we address potential nutritional deficiencies on an all-plant diet? According to Dr. John McDougall, since the usual dietary source of vitamin B_{12} for carnivores and some omnivores is the flesh of other animals, the obvious conclusion is that those who choose to avoid eating meat are destined to become B_{12} deficient. There is a grain of truth in this concern, but in reality that rarely happens to any otherwise healthy strict vegetarian. Since the amount of B_{12} required in a lifetime is the equivalent of less than the weight of three grains of rice (that's micrograms per day), Dr. McDougall states that the chances of deficiency are one in a million. In fact, he says that people who come into their program with deficiencies find that, after subsequent blood tests, their deficiencies will be reduced or eliminated by the plant-based diet.

Those people who are concerned about getting the essential vitamins found in abundance in meats can consider two possibilities for supplementation of B_{12} and also D_3. Our digestive tracts produce a minute amount of B_{12}, probably not enough to suffice, so we suggest a sublingual form of B_{12} that will provide about 250 milligrams per week. Our bodies also manufacture the D hormone, but because of lack of sunlight and the inefficiency of the D that is present in pasteurized milk, a D_3 supplement (providing about 5,000 IUs per day) can be extremely helpful. Another possible deficiency is the omega fats, prevalent in fish oils but also in some plants. Supplements that are natural, such as raw flaxseed, hemp powder, or chia seed, are some of the highest, most efficient forms of organic omega fatty acids. You can take whole raw flaxseed or chia seed, put it in a small electric coffee grinder, and make a fine powder. Put it in your freezer, and every week take a heaping tablespoon and add it to a drink or a salad.

GETTING RESULTS

So you see that you can accomplish dramatic weight loss and that this can be accomplished largely without an arsenal of supplemental vitamins. On the Birchcreek program hypertension, high blood pressure, and heart disease are reduced, diminished, or eliminated. Type 2 diabetics who were dependent on medicines and injections tell us great, miraculous success stories. People find that acid reflux and allergies disappear very, very quickly.

Sleeping disorders take from two weeks to a month to be replaced with normal sleep patterns. We have had people stay with us for one to two weeks who had not had a restful night's sleep in twenty years. Before they leave, they testify that they have just had the soundest, most refreshing night sleep, night after night, that they had experienced in years.

On this diet cholesterol levels return to normal levels. We have people who have been on blood thinners to prevent blood clots or stroke. People who come to the program are required to have regular blood tests, weekly or biweekly, to monitor changes in their blood. It is a long process that can take up to a month to see significant reductions in natural blood thinning, but the program provides a one-way street to normal.

If you don't process nutrition adequately from the food you consume, your doctor may have prescribed supplements and vitamins for you. In some rare cases these will still be needed, because the person's body is not performing normally. But be careful not to assume that your body is incapable of getting nutrition. It may be that your diet has consisted of such narrow choices that you have simply missed vital nutrients from foods.

After one month on a quality high-octane, broad, plant-based diet, a person's body reaches a level where we can ascertain if a supplement is required. So before you resort to supplements, you might consider broadening your diet. If your blood work continues to exhibit deficiencies, then perhaps you should consider supplementation to remedy those deficiencies.

Often, overall health hinges on the absorption and metabolism of calcium. Calcium pills and calcium-rich foods may be delivering calcium in the wrong form. You need to be aware of the conditions that create favorable calcium absorption:

- Calcium-rich foods should be consumed raw so as to maintain the active enzyme associated with helping the efficient absorption of calcium. When calcium-rich foods are cooked, the bonded enzyme is destroyed, and the breakdown and absorption of calcium are severely diminished.

- Sound sleep is required for the completion of the reconstruction of the skeleton. Deep sleep cycles provide the best opportunity for the body to rebuild bone, ligaments, and tendons. In general sleep is a symbiotic necessity, serving to restore, rejuvenate, and recalibrate the body's biological systems.

- Consuming quality vitamin C is needed to maintain the solubility of calcium and to help absorb it into the bloodstream. Good sources are oranges, other citrus fruits, and avocadoes. An avocado has about six times the vitamin C potency of an orange. Without vitamin C all the other good things you have done to get calcium into your system will fall short.

- Vitamin D is another important cornerstone in the metabolism and absorption of calcium. Without ample D it doesn't matter how many calcium-rich foods you eat. D is a hormone that is vital to calcium absorption. Currently calcium intake recommendations are not directly associated with vitamin D status, which may explain why markedly different recommended calcium intakes exist among countries. In the United States, the recommended calcium intake is 1,200 milligrams (mg) daily for adults aged fifty and older. D is the hormone that cows produce by grazing in the grass under the sun, and it can be obtained by drinking their milk. There is just as much D in milk as ever, but the milk we drink has been fortified with vitamin D because we aren't getting enough.

ENOUGH ABOUT VITAMINS!

How can a society that spends in excess of five billion dollars a year on vitamins claim any good from vitamins?[10] The people taking those supplements are the same people who are suffering from the same types and rates of illness as the general population. Vitamins and supplements have become big business. Advertisers tell us that our bodies require certain vitamins in order to achieve proper health and function and their product supplies that very need. The confidence attained by taking pills instead of eating properly seems to reassure people in the same way that an insurance policy does. But vitamins alone can't guarantee health.

Many people who visit our facilities are heavy vitamin users and yet experience the same full range of degenerative diseases and maladies as the rest of the American population. Birchcreek clients suspend their supplemental vitamin regimen and adopt a raw, plant-based diet. As they invariably and dramatically lose weight and improve their health, many never need to go back to the supplements. Someone who had taken vitamins for years once said to me, after experiencing better health with our program, "With all the money I spent on vitamins, I was making very expensive urine!" So remember, eat a wide variety of high-octane foods first to improve your weight and health. Give your system about a month to balance, cleanse, detox, and improve itself. Then test for deficiencies and supplement where necessary.

CHAPTER 18

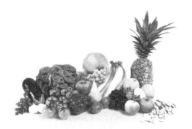

PRACTICAL, NOT PERFECT— LIFE IN TRANSITION

t may seem unreasonable to expect all the people who want to enhance their health and lose weight to read this book, to go "cold turkey"—pardon the pun—and give up meat and dairy altogether. As Eddie Rivera (the wilderness hiking guide at Birchcreek) would say, "What hill do you want to die on?"

How much can you eliminate? Can you eliminate meat and dairy only part of the time and still gain nutritional benefits? How can you accommodate occasional meals containing meat or dairy?

You have some tough decisions to make. The Baby Boomer generation, Generation Xers, Millennials, and all the rest of us have been weaned on meat and dairy. We can never escape the history of our dietary culture and the marketing techniques of the twenty-first century. The fast-food commercials and the beautiful people wearing white milk mustaches are ubiquitous. Meat and dairy are so much a part of our culture that it does seem impossible to reduce or eliminate animal products even if you have become convinced that you should.

KNOW YOUR MINIMUM GOALS BEFORE YOU BEGIN

What is your goal? To eat more healthily? To lose weight? To diminish your probability of heart disease or cancer? Most certainly you are aiming to improve something if you have been reading this book.

Eating higher-octane foods while decreasing your consumption of low-octane foods is basically the path to the improvement you seek. For those, and there will be many, who enjoy their meat and dairy and are not willing to stop, but who are willing to dramatically reduce their consumption of animal products, let me say this: you can lose weight and get healthier by restricting the frequency and type of animal products you eat, provided that you consume copious amounts of plant food while you are consuming fewer animal products.

Certain types of fish, both raw and cooked, are less harmful than others and offer some benefit if consumed far less frequently than recommended by standard American nutritional advisors. Sardines and cold-water fish such as natural salmon, trout, tuna, mackerel, cod, or bluefish are high in omegas and are considered a good way to meet certain nutritional needs. Bottom-dwelling fish, however, along with shellfish, swordfish, shark, and most other fish are far less beneficial for humans. Transitioning to a once-a-week consumption of one of the healthier fish choices instead of other meats would bring significant improvement in health.

Meats other than fish are far less forgiving. Processed meats such as ham, bologna, salami, or any other deli-type cold cuts should never be consumed—by anybody.

But understand that there are far safer plant foods containing virtually all of the same nutrition benefits without the harmful downside of having animal products in your system. Substitutes such as seeds from the chia plant or carefully processed hemp protein powder contain superior omega fatty acids and protein.

SOME FAQS

Q. If I choose to eat meat, dairy, and other processed foods, how much and how often can I eat them without harming my health or reintroducing more toxicity?

A. The answer lies in some of the formulas that explain how long animal products take to successfully pass through our digestive tracts. Animal products take from seventy-two to ninety hours to pass out of our systems. That's between three and four days. So naturally we should at least try to transition into eating animal products slightly longer than seventy-two to ninety hours apart, ideally no more than every four or five days.

Q. I would assume portion control is important when consuming seafood. What can you tell us about this?

A. Small portions, no larger than a deck of playing cards, are highly recommended. A large raw leafy salad should precede the meal. Water, a wonderful detoxifier, should be your beverage of choice. With all meals, but especially with those featuring meat and seafood, a habit of eating a salad first should be cemented into your regimen.

Q. What is more harmful—meat, dairy, or fish?

A. All animal products offer nutritional benefits, but animal products also create unhealthy by-products. I consider cow's milk to be far more harmful than red meat and fish to be less harmful than red meats. Again, I believe that a limited consumption of select fish is not bad.

Q. If I want to just lose weight, why should I be interested in reducing or eliminating meat and dairy?

A. Weight loss is a function of metabolizing stores of fat and reconverting this into energy. This transaction requires more calories to be burned than the number that will sustain your current weight. This dynamic exchange is regulated by diet and activity. When you are trying to lose weight simply by adjusting the standard American diet, you are starving your body of nutrition. This condition places your autonomic system in survival mode, and your body stingily allows as little fat as possible to be converted into energy. We have heard it before in these words: "You have a slow metabolism." The trick is to rev up your metabolism with high-octane foods and physical activity. As your chemistry changes, your metabolism responds accordingly. Your body will facilitate the translation from fat to glucose in a far more efficient way. With the chemistry of your body optimized, fat is readily converted to glucose, driving your energy level through the roof. This represents biological momentum in the right direction.

Q. Can I sustain a healthy diet if I radically reduce my intake of meat?

A. You are really asking how you can transition so as not to sabotage your long-term success. Those who chose not to eliminate animal products from their diets can still dramatically improve their health, weight, and longevity. By following our guidelines, you can assist your own body to achieve success. How closely you follow our program will determine how permanently your change will last.

WEIGHT LOSS ALONE ... NOT ENOUGH

Meat and dairy are getting pretty badly beaten up lately. But even when you believe what many health and weight-loss books are saying about animal products, you may not be quite ready, or you may never be ready, to completely give up meat, dairy, or an occasional New York strip steak.

If this is you, you must ask yourself, "What are my goals?" And they should be *goals* plural, not *goal* singular. Why? Because it is like fool's gold to try to achieve mere weight loss without knowing the best way to lose weight or detoxing without nourishing your body. We get excited about fasting and losing five or ten pounds, while the prize yields no long-term dividends. In other words, most shortcuts are dead ends. Even if you were to miraculously wake up tomorrow morning as fit and energetic as you would like to be, how do you presume you would maintain this?

Practical, not perfect is the key phrase. Transition is the methodology. If you are trying to eliminate, reduce, or extinguish bad eating habits or unhealthy cravings, or develop a resolve to conquer compulsions, transitioning the Birchcreek way offers the best opportunity to succeed.

HEALTHY EATING WITH PLEASURE RATHER THAN EATING FOR PLEASURE

We all would like to wake up the finished product. But it just doesn't happen that way. Usually it is a journey, a transition. Resolving to make a change is usually fueled through willpower, and yet willpower alone is not the answer we expect it to be. In fact, willpower may not be an integral part in your success at all. I do believe it is part of the process. But your success should never depend on whether you think you have enough willpower or not.

Historically a crisis arrives when a willpower-driven diet crashes head-on into your cravings for those tasty bad foods you have been eating for years. And when your will to eat healthy capitulates to your desire for satisfying taste, you throw your hands up and say, "This is impossible!" Well, you are right. Willpower is temporary and short-lived.

It is not about willpower. I know what you're thinking. Even the thought of changing your diet permanently seems daunting for the average person. Most solutions offered are shortcuts. So let me state the facts. There are no shortcuts. You cannot sustain a lifelong change by using willpower alone. So what's the answer? I express it with a trio of ideas:

1. Introduction

2. Accommodation

3. Nesting

Introduction

First, allow yourself new food encounters that are healthy and taste great. Concerning meat, choose a better type of meat. Always try to improve your choices; it goes a long way to permanently changing your diet. Also realize that what you put on your meat is oftentimes why you enjoy it. Dressings and sauces for meat are usually harmful to your health. See if you can improve your choices, looking for more natural accompaniments. Try new tastes. If you go ahead and eliminate some of your favorite meat dressings, you might eat less meat over the long haul.

Accommodation

Next, begin to indulge in the new foods and tastes that you kind of like or even love. This means setting up times or circumstances to enjoy that new food even more. From there let your perfectly reliable brain do the rest.

Nesting

This is what happens when you begin to acquire a taste for something. Don't worry! Just as you created habits and cravings regarding all your other foods, so will you now create new habits. Eating a healthier choice of meat or fish, flavoring it with a more natural dressing, along with a regimen of large, leafy salad before your main course will soon become your new normal. Again, it is important to sequence the consumption of animal products four to five days apart.

As a side note in developing healthier diets, we should be so lucky as to reach the compulsion stage of eating healthy foods. Reaching the craving stage of healthy eating is expected and will occur if you make a systematic plan. That is how you acquired your habits, cravings, and compulsions in the first place. It doesn't upset the apple cart to follow these guidelines.

Remember the three necessities:

1. Never sacrifice your taste or taste-driven decisions.

2. Remember "octane," and choose foods in their most natural form.

3. Make sure of your ability to buy food at an ordinary grocery or shopping center—that's called accessibility.

WHAT ABOUT WILLPOWER?

Thus, you can see how your willpower is needed but not as the driving force to success. Instead you can regard your willpower as the pilot light to your engine. Your engine is your desire to finally make a significant change in your weight, health, and vitality. The pilot light remains lit as the starting point in your transition as you learn to trust your autonomic response to developing new, pleasurable food-related habits that will drive themselves.

The introduction and repetition of new food choices will grow on you, naturally and without much fanfare. As they do, they automatically begin to dovetail into your eating regimen. Your brain will begin to develop affection for this once-new food you introduced to your family of foods, and you will find yourself on the road to better health.

WHAT DOES PROGRESS LOOK LIKE?

Shifting food choices by reducing consumption of some foods while increasing consumption of others is the primary strategy for most successful dietary transitions. By using this method, you can control the munchies, in a sense putting out the fires of unhealthy cravings one by one. This method is the opposite of cold turkey and offers a person a doable approach to maintaining weight loss, increasing energy reserves, and continuing to reduce toxins. At the biochemical level, the transaction from high-octane nutrition to energy accelerates, while the production of waste goes down. How far you are willing to go will depend on you—and how well you feel will translate into more resolve to undertake new levels of transition. Your tastes will be broader than before. This higher-octane food will blunt cravings while the new tastes satisfy at the most superficial level. Never give up eating for taste. It is already programmed in. Go ahead and be superficial. Use it!

THE ONE-TWO-THREE PUNCH

"Practical, not perfect" is a methodology that most people can embrace. Whether or not you are additionally motivated by vanity or illness, this approach works. If you are driven by a desire to look as good as you can for yourself or the one you love, or you are striving to achieve a longer, healthier life, this method works. More importantly, there is no disqualification in how long it might take.

Deliver the first one-two-three punch combination to begin. Your first bite into high-octane food and your first reduction or elimination of dangerous foods begins the transition.

The following diagram may be helpful in aligning your ambition to your expectations. The closer you are to the center, the more rapid your weight loss and detoxification. Begin to develop a vision of how progress looks. You may not ever eliminate meat or dairy from your diet completely. But believing in the natural science of how your mind and body works best and putting faith in this system can dramatically improve the journey.

THE ONE-TWO-THREE PUNCH

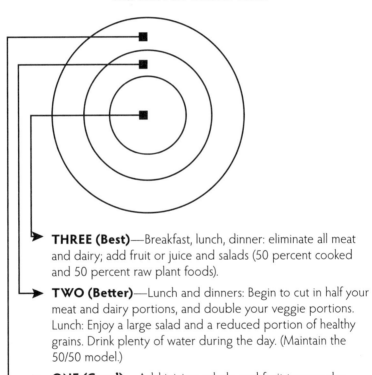

THREE (Best)—Breakfast, lunch, dinner: eliminate all meat and dairy; add fruit or juice and salads (50 percent cooked and 50 percent raw plant foods).

TWO (Better)—Lunch and dinners: Begin to cut in half your meat and dairy portions, and double your veggie portions. Lunch: Enjoy a large salad and a reduced portion of healthy grains. Drink plenty of water during the day. (Maintain the 50/50 model.)

ONE (Good)—Add juicing, salads, and fruit to your day, especially for breakfast and snacks. This in itself will begin to ruin a poor diet. Satisfy tastes and cravings with new foods such as raw nuts, seeds, smoothies, fresh sorbets, hummus, veggies, and healthy dips with healthy chips. (You will begin to notice how much easier it is to portion-control your treats.)

BE VERSATILE

Your course is set. The tide is right. You set sail immediately. In the past you have tried everything, procrastinated, explored, reeducated yourself, and practically jumped through hoops attempting to lose weight or regain your health and vitality. It is time to set a course and let your autopilot autonomic system take you to the finish line. You need a course you can follow without adding extra crew or high-tech equipment.

You have everything you need to set sail with full expectation of arriving successfully. It is not uncharted territory. Birchcreek's diet plan works virtually 100 percent of the time when people just apply the knowledge and understanding derived from this book. Oh, yes—you must take along the provision of *faith*. Before now you have put so much faith in portion control, counting protein, counting carbs, counting calories, and so forth. How about putting faith in your miraculous human body? It was created for such a time as this. How it works is miraculous, and how it responds to opportunity is as dependable as you would expect from the highest form of life on earth.

You may find at times that "tacking" is appropriate. As a sailing enthusiast and sailboat owner, I know firsthand that getting from point A to point B may require some back and forth. The shortest distance may not always be a straight line. Changing your dietary lifestyle happens with ebb and flow much like sailing. You will encounter winds, tides, and currents. You measure your progress very differently than you would in a straight-line race.

If sailing teaches us anything about competing, it teaches that there is more than one way to compete. There may be different results achieved by different people traveling the same path, even the same tack. Anytime you are not satisfied with how your vessel handles in a particular wind or circumstance, you can make a course correction. You are unique.

Our machines run on the same fuel and respond in the same basic ways. But there are always exceptions to the rule. Severe allergies, digestive disorders, unresponsiveness to certain food types, and necessary medications can demand a specialized diet. What works for someone in Florida may not work for someone in Ohio. Different cultures, jobs, lifestyles, circumstances, financial abilities, and health are the winds and currents that sometimes blow us off course or demand tweaking of our tack.

But with faith as your provision, you can maintain your course. You can be assured of the finish line because you know how your own vessel runs best.

Take the helm! Set sail immediately.

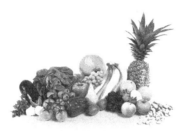

FINAL WORD

You will begin to notice, on your new journey, a vast array of colors, textures, aromas, and flavors. If you take one of our Birchcreek cooking classes, we can teach you how to mix color and texture, thereby deriving a wide range of nutrition. Just think about the cornucopia of fruits and vegetables and all of the plant foods that come out of this earth. They are far more attractive than a steak or a glass of milk. The colors and flavors of natural foods are like the colors of a rainbow, and their aromas are tantalizing.

As you detoxify your body, you will be cleansing your sensory faculties and boosting the sensitivity of your receptors. You will enable your tongue and your palate to taste and appreciate the subtleties and the extravagant bursts of flavor from living foods. Just as a wine taster appreciates the character of wine, so you too will begin to appreciate your new-found ability to discern tastes. A discerning eater enjoys and appreciates tastes and can distinguish between many.

Now that food is no longer in control of you, eating can become a pleasure, a joy, and a hobby. Have fun! Host food parties! Be the social director who introduces your friends to food combinations that you have designed with your creativity. Bring along with you as many as will follow, so in your old age you won't have lost friends to unnecessary disease.

THE SEVEN GIFTS TO LASTING HEALTH

As a final reminder, here are the topics that hold your most important keys to success. They provide miraculous change.

1. Food, living food is the first and foremost weapon against obesity and disease. Incorporate large glasses of fresh juice with your solid food diet.

2. Pure water hydrates and detoxifies the body. You need to drink plenty of water, preferably not municipal water. Two gallons a day is not too much.

3. Sunlight is good for you, in moderation. Take a daily walk; get out in the sun.

4. Exercise is good for you too—not exercise that breaks your body or taxes the limits of your skeleton or your muscle structure, but moderate exercise. You can do moderate exercise for the rest of your life, regardless of

age, to keep your body toned, fit, agile, and responsive.

5. Proper rest calibrates your body clock, refocuses your mind, and regenerates the tissues of your body.

6. Emotional balance is not something you can plan, but if everything else in this list is in order, you are going to be emotionally sound. Your brain is subject to the chemistry of your body.

7. Spiritual grounding gives you relevance and purpose. It reassures you that you are important and unique. You have been designed for a long healthy life. The Bible tells you that you have been made in the very image of God (Genesis 1:26–27); that you are wonderfully made, and all the days of your life were written in God's book before you were even born (Psalm 139:13–16); that you were chosen before the foundations of the earth were formed (Ephesians 1:4); and that you are God's own possession, that you have an inheritance in Him, and that you were chosen for the praise of His glory (Ephesians 1:13–14).

KNOWLEDGE—WITH UNDERSTANDING AND WISDOM

We can change our lives, our health, and our weight for good. That's what the proper application of this knowledge can do for us. This book should serve as a commonsense guide for applying what you have learned about your miraculous human body. Humans may be the only creatures on earth who cook their food, but it happens to be a pleasant and possibly a necessary evil to maintain our sanity. Most people who succeed in transitioning to a plant-based diet settle into a pattern or ratio of 50 percent raw to 50 percent cooked. That's practical, and practical habits can last a lifetime—a long lifetime!

Appendix A

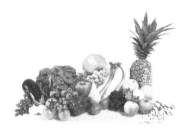

BIRCHCREEK JUICE FAST

by Julie Odato

The term *juicing* means the extraction of fresh juices from raw fruits, vegetables, and greens, usually using an electric kitchen juicer or blender, but sometimes using a hand citrus-juicer. After the juicing process, there are two end products—liquids and fiber. The addition of the concentrated nutrition of fresh juices to a diet increases vegetable intake and helps the body's immune system. Juicing is an ideal way to improve the diets of children.

Juice fasting means drinking only raw fresh juices for a prescribed period of time. Juice fasting is considered an excellent cleanse or "detox" catalyst for the human body. Besides juice, most juice fasts include large amounts of water and/or herbal (caffeine-free) teas. After a specified length of time, juice fasting is followed by a return to eating. Immediately following a fast, we recommend a day of eating only raw fruits and vegetables. During the week following a fast, we tell people to consume plenty of raw fruits and vegetables daily, with a cooked vegetarian entrée (including whole grains) in the evening for dinner.

A *juice cleanse* is a program designed to reduce concentrated toxins, preservatives, and pesticides in the body while increasing consumption of clean, healthy, whole nutrients in order to facilitate internal cleansing and accelerated weight loss. Always check with your doctor before starting this or any diet plan.

During a juice fast or a juice cleanse, people may continue all prescribed medications unless otherwise recommended by a doctor. However, nutritional supplements should be suspended during a juice fast unless prescribed by a doctor. Hydration is important during a juice fast—you should drink at least 48 ounces of water or caffeine-free tea daily in addition to the juices.

When they undertake a juice fast, most people report experiencing few or none of the following symptoms. If symptoms do appear, it is usually in the first three or four days of beginning a fast. All symptoms are temporary. If they persist or are severe, please return to eating and consult with your health care professional. Feel free to take your normal pain reliever if necessary.

- Mild headache
- Lethargy

- Moodiness

- Skin breakout

- Tongue coating

- Change in skin scent

- Feeling cold

- Nausea

- Flu-like symptoms

What about physical activity during a juice fast? Most people are able to function physically as normal during a juice fast or a juice cleanse. We recommend at least forty-five minutes of brisk walking daily, with or without hand free weights, depending upon your physical ability.

TEN-DAY JUICE FAST

- All ingredients are juiced together in a juicer (not a blender) or a citrus juicer.

- All breakfast juices are 8 ounces for women and 16 ounces for men. All lunch and dinner juices are 16 ounces.

- Drink a powdered green shot thirty minutes before breakfast each day.*

- Drink citrus water midmorning between breakfast and lunch (sliced orange, lemon, lime, and grapefruit in a glass of water, slightly chilled).

---

* We recommend BarleyMax (available online).

- Drink organic vegan veggie broth or bouillon midafternoon daily.**
- Add a 1 tablespoon of natural hemp protein powder or chia seed powder to water or juices daily to ensure adequate protein intake.***
- All fruits and vegetables should be organic, if possible. Otherwise, scrub or peel.

Day 1

- *Breakfast:* Fresh Citrus (2 navel oranges, ½ pink grapefruit, 1 lemon, 1 lime)
- *Lunch:* Tomato (7 medium plum tomatoes)
- *Dinner:* Salad in a Glass (1 beefsteak tomato, 1 large peeled cucumber, 1 stalk celery, ½ green pepper, 5 green leaf lettuce leaves, dash of vinegar)

Day 2

- *Breakfast:* Apple-Blueberry (3 apples, ⅓ cup blueberries)
- *Lunch:* Banana Mango Smoothie (1 frozen ripe banana, ½ cup frozen mango, ½ cup unsweetened rice or almond milk, combined in blender)
- *Dinner:* Orange Parade (7 ounces organic pumpkin, 1 large unpeeled sweet potato, ¼

** We recommend Rapunzel brand vegan vegetable bouillon cubes (available online or in health food stores).

*** Available in health food stores.

navel orange, ½ pound California juicing carrots)

Day 3

- *Breakfast:* Pear Kiwi (4 Anjou pears, 1 unpeeled kiwi)

- *Lunch:* Green Apple (5 green Granny Smith apples, 1 stalk broccoli, ½ green pepper, ⅛ head green cabbage, 4 spinach leaves, 4 stalks parsley)

- *Dinner:* Carrot Ginger (2 pounds California juicing carrots, ½-inch piece of ginger)

Day 4

- *Breakfast:* Melon Madness (2-inch wedge of cantaloupe, three-inch wedge of watermelon)

- *Lunch:* Smoothie (½ cup unsweetened almond milk, ½ cup frozen raspberries, 6 frozen large strawberries, water to blend)

- *Dinner:* Salsa (6 medium Roma tomatoes, ½ green bell pepper, ¼ red pepper, ⅛ small onion, 2 6-inch stalks cilantro, ⅛ clove garlic)

Day 5

- *Breakfast:* Pear Grape (4 pears, 10 red or green grapes)

- *Lunch:* Pink Lady (1 pineapple, trimmed and peeled; ⅛ head red cabbage; 2 McIntosh apples)

- *Dinner:* Guacamole in a Glass (1 avocado, 4 medium plum tomatoes, juice of 1 lime)

Day 6

- *Breakfast:* Fresh Citrus (2 navel oranges, ½ pink grapefruit)
- *Lunch:* Banana Calmer (1 banana, 12 ounces unsweetened almond milk, ⅛ teaspoon cinnamon, ¼ teaspoon vanilla extract, combined in a blender)
- *Dinner:* Carrot (2 pounds of carrots, scrubbed)

Day 7

- *Breakfast:* Apple Beet (3 McIntosh apples, ½ small raw beet)
- *Lunch:* Cranberry Carrot (2 pounds carrots, ¼ cup cranberries)
- *Dinner:* Green Machine (1 head green lettuce leaves, 8 stalks parsley, 2 stalks celery, ¼ pound spinach, 2 green apples)

Day 8

- *Breakfast:* Carrot (1 pound carrots, scrubbed)
- *Lunch:* Red Bull (3 medium tomatoes, 1 red bell pepper, ¼ teaspoon hot sauce)
- *Dinner:* Cucumber Kiwi (2 large peeled cucumbers, 2 kiwis, ¼ lime)

Day 9

- *Breakfast:* Pear Ginger (4 pears, sliver of ginger)
- *Lunch:* Citrus Veggie (1 pound carrots, 2 oranges, ½ lemon, 4 leaves green leafy lettuce, 1 stalk broccoli)
- *Dinner:* Tomato Zinger Cocktail (4 medium tomatoes, 1 cup beet greens, 3 radishes)

Day 10

- *Breakfast:* Apple Mint (4 crisp apples, 1 sprig fresh mint, 1 sprig parsley)
- *Lunch:* Smoothie (1 cup unsweetened almond milk, ½ cup frozen peaches, 1 cup frozen strawberries, water to blend)
- *Dinner:* It's Italian (3 medium tomatoes, 1 stalk broccoli rabe, ¼ small clove garlic, ¼ cup fresh basil leaves)

APPENDIX B

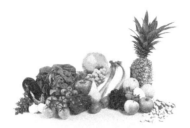

BIRCHCREEK RECIPES

compiled by Julie Odato

Before you start on the Jump-Start Your Life diet, you will need to make some changes in your kitchen and pantry. For starters, remove ancient bottles of seasoning, beef and chicken bouillon, and processed and prepared foods. Replace coffee with organic decaf, or better yet, herbal teas and Postum or another grain beverage. Get rid of all artificial sweeteners, nondairy creamer products, canned goods with added sugar and preservatives, and boxed cake mixes, muffin mixes, and so forth. Replace your canned goods with frozen or fresh items, buying what is in season whenever possible. Replace soda and sweetened drinks (including artificially sweetened water) with

217

flavored water, without sweeteners, and herbal or decaf iced tea sweetened with honey. Or start drinking plain, pure water.

Then revise your recipes. Go through your favorite recipes and see if the harmful ingredients can be replaced by less harmful ones. For example, replace white sugar with honey or maple syrup, white flour with the whole-grain flour, white pasta with whole-grain pasta, and so on. Remember that whole-grain foods should be kept in the freezer to prevent spoilage.

THE BIRCHCREEK PANTRY

One of the secrets to your success is having the proper items on hand in your kitchen. When the urge to snack or cook hits you, reach for natural whole foods instead of processed junk. The following is a short list of some necessary staples:

- Whole-grain pasta (including spinach, rice, whole wheat, corn, udon pastas)
- Rice (brown rice, brown basmati rice, wild rice)—to replace white rice
- Couscous (whole grain)—excellent as a side dish or in a combination of vegetables
- Whole-wheat flour—replaces white flour (keep it in the freezer)
- Celtic Sea Salt—sun-dried, contains all naturally occurring elements with no added chemicals
- Herb seasoning—usually found in health food stores

- Lemon juice—can be used in place of vinegar for a different flavor

GROCERY SHOPPING

Some good products to keep on hand include the following:

- Vegenaise—our favorite commercial mayonnaise replacement

- Brown mustard—excellent for seasoning and salad dressings

- Arrowroot powder—used as a thickener in place of cornstarch

- Sweeteners—raw honey, pure maple syrup, molasses, apple juice, stevia

- Tahini—ground sesame seed/olive oil paste

- Tamari—used instead of soy sauce

- Balsamic, apple cider, wine vinegar—for salad dressing recipes

- Raw sunflower, pumpkin, sesame seeds— usually must be bought in a health food store to guarantee raw

- Raisins—usually must be bought in a health food store to guarantee organic

- Raw flaxseed oil, olive oil, or Udos Choice perfected oil blend—hydrogenated oils

- Extra-virgin olive oil—best oil to use for dressing or food preparation

- Milk—almond milk, rice milk, or sunflower milk (all unsweetened)

FRUIT JUICE RECIPES

Mixed fruit juice combinations (1 serving)

Use about five hard apples (like McIntosh) and a handful of berries or a few chunks of other fruits to make the following combinations:

- Apple Cranberry
- Apple Pear
- Apple Mango
- Apple Cherry
- Apple Grape
- Apple Strawberry
- Apple Blueberry
- Apple Watermelon
- Apple Pineapple
- Apple Raspberry

Other fruit combinations (1 serving)

- Pineapple Peach (1 whole pineapple, 1 peach)
- Pineapple Grapefruit (1 pineapple, 1 grapefruit)
- Pineapple Citrus (1 pineapple, 1 orange, 1 lemon)
- Pineapple Kiwi (1 pineapple, 2 kiwis)
- Pineapple Pear (1 pineapple, 1 pear)
- Pineapple Coconut (1 pineapple, ¼ cup organic canned milk)
- Grapefruit Orange (1 grapefruit, 3 oranges)
- Strawberry Peach (3 peaches, 5 strawberries)

- Cranberry Orange Lemon (3 oranges, ¼ cup cranberries, 1 lemon)

Fruit-veggie combos (1 serving)

- Pineapple Red Cabbage (1 pineapple, 2 green or red apples, ¼ cup red cabbage)
- Pineapple Celery (1 pineapple, 1 green apple, 1 stalk celery)
- Grapefruit Cucumber (1 cucumber, 1 grapefruit)
- Apple Broccoli (5 apples, 2 stalks broccoli)
- Orange Carrot Ginger (1 lb. carrots, 1 orange, sliver ginger)
- Apple Fennel Cucumber (2 apples, 1 cucumber, ⅛ cup fennel)
- Apple Beet (5 green apples, ½ small beet)
- Apple Carrot (1 lb. carrots, 2 crisp apples)
- Pineapple Lettuce Cilantro (1 pineapple, 3 lettuce leaves, 2 stalks cilantro)
- Pineapple Carrot (½ pineapple, 1 lb. carrots)
- Orange Cucumber (1 cucumber, 2 oranges)

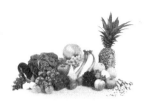

VEGETABLE JUICE RECIPES

Each of the following juice recipes is one serving.

RED BELL PEPPER BOOSTER

1 cup carrot juice

1 cup tomato juice

2 large red bell peppers

1 Tbsp. lemon juice

ORANGE SURPRISE

1 sweet potato

¼ cup pumpkin

1 cup carrot juice

¼ cup orange juice

Dash nutmeg, cinnamon, or pumpkin pie spice

GINGER CRUSH

1 cup carrot juice

4 tomatoes

1 Tbsp. lemon juice

Sliver of fresh ginger root

Tomato "Soup"

    5 tomatoes
    1 avocado
    1 Tbsp. sea salt

Celery Surprise

    ½ cup carrot juice
    4 tomatoes
    3 celery stalks
    4 scallions
    Handful fresh parsley

Italian Tomato

    7 plum tomatoes
    ⅓ green pepper
    1 clove garlic
    ¼ small onion
    Handful fresh basil

Green Goddess

    5 apples
    1 green pepper
    Few stalks of cilantro

Tiger Tom

    2 plum tomatoes
    1 carrot
    ½ jalapeño pepper

SALSA

5 tomatoes

1 clove garlic

2 stalks cilantro

1 green pepper

Juice of 1 lime

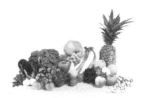

SALAD RECIPES

||||||||||||||||||||||||||||||||||||||||||||||||||||||||||||||||||||||||||||||||||||||||||||||||

AVOCADO TOMATO SALAD

2 cups diced tomatoes

1 cup fresh basil, chopped

½ cup olive oil

1 cup Maui onion (or red onion), chopped

1 Tbsp. fresh oregano

⅓ cup lemon juice

1½ tsp. Celtic Sea Salt

1 Tbsp. black olives, chopped

1 cup cubed avocado

Combine ingredients in a large bowl. Mix and serve over lettuce. *Serves 4.*

||||||||||||||||||||||||||||||||||||||||||||||||||||||||||||||||||||||||||||||||||||||||||||

WALDORF SALAD

4–5 large apples, cored and chunked

½ cup walnuts

½ cup raisins

2 stalks celery, chopped

1 Tbsp. lemon juice

Dash sea salt

Vegenaise, to taste

Mix together all ingredients and coat with Vegenaise. Chill before serving. *Serves 4.*

||||||||||||||||||||||||||||||||||||||||||||||||||||||||||||||||||||||||||||||||||||

SUMMER LEAF AND HERB SALAD

> Inner leaves from 2 large romaine lettuce hearts
> 8 oz. mixed salad leaves, such as radicchio,
> mizuna, or endive
> Handful of mixed, fresh, soft-leaf herbs such as
> basil, chives, dill, and mint

Wash the salad leaves, spin dry in a salad spinner (or pat dry with paper towels), and transfer to a plastic bag. Chill for 30 minutes to make the leaves crisp.

Put the leaves and herbs in a large salad bowl, add a little of the dressing, and toss well to coat evenly. Add a little more dressing to taste then serve. (Best served with Honey Lemon Dressing.) *Serves 2.*

||||||||||||||||||||||||||||||||||||||||||||||||||||||||||||||||||||||||||||||||||||

APPLE/CABBAGE HOLIDAY SLAW

> ½ medium-sized head green cabbage,
> shredded
> 1 cup organic raisins
> 4 apples, peeled and shredded
> ½ cup unsweetened coconut, shredded
> (optional)
> Juice from 2 apples
> ½ cup fresh lemon juice
> ¼ cup honey
> Pumpkin pie spice, to taste

Mix all ingredients together and refrigerate till mealtime. *Serves 4.*

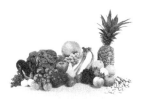

SALAD DRESSING RECIPES

HONEY LEMON DRESSING

1 garlic clove, crushed
½ cup extra-virgin olive oil
1 Tbsp. freshly squeezed lemon juice
1 tsp. honey
1 tsp. Dijon mustard
Sea salt and freshly ground black pepper,
to taste

Put the dressing ingredients in a bowl or small jug and set aside to infuse for at least 1 hour. Just before serving, strain out the garlic. *Serves 4.*

GINGER DRESSING

4 cloves garlic
4 Tbsp. ginger
½ cup olive oil
⅔ cup rice vinegar
1 cup tamari
¼ cup honey
2 cups water

Place all ingredients in blender and blend until smooth. Store in a glass jar, covered, in the refrigerator. Dressing can be placed in warm water to loosen honey. Shake well before serving. *Serves 4.*

||||||||||||||||||||||||||||||||||||||||||||||||||||||||||||||||||||||||||||||||

BALSAMIC VINAIGRETTE

⅔ cup extra-virgin olive oil
⅓ cup balsamic vinegar
1 Tbsp. chopped leeks
1 Tbsp. fresh basil
2 tsp. fresh thyme
1 tsp. raw honey
Celtic Sea Salt, to taste

Place all ingredients in blender and blend until smooth. *Serves 6.*

||||||||||||||||||||||||||||||||||||||||||||||||||||||||||||||||||||||||||||||||

COLESLAW DRESSING

1 cup apple cider vinegar
1 cup extra-virgin olive oil
1 Tbsp. raw honey
1 clove garlic
Celtic Sea Salt, to taste

Place all ingredients in blender and blend until smooth. *Serves 6.*

||||||||||||||||||||||||||||||||||||||||||||||||||||||||||||||||||||||||||||||||

CREAMY RANCH DRESSING

1 cup water
1 cup almonds
1 tsp. basil
1 tsp. onion flakes or powder

½ tsp. garlic powder

1 tsp. raw honey

3 Tbsp. fresh lemon juice

Celtic Sea Salt, to taste

Blend water and almonds in blender until smooth. Remove from blender. Stir in remaining ingredients. Chill and serve. *Serves 4.*

ITALIAN CAESAR DRESSING

2 Tbsp. extra-virgin olive oil

¼ tsp. parsley

¼ tsp. oregano

¼ tsp. basil

(or use 1 tsp. of Italian seasoning instead of parsley, oregano, and basil)

½ capful apple cider vinegar

¼ tsp. Vegenaise

Celtic Sea Salt, to taste

Place all ingredients in blender and blend until smooth. Chill and serve. *Serves 1.*

MANGO DRESSING

1 ripe mango

1 Tbsp. fresh ginger, minced

¼ cup fresh apple juice or water

Place all ingredients in blender and blend until smooth. *Serves 2.*

SUNFLOWER DRESSING

1½ cups sunflower seeds
2 cups water
½ cup fresh lemon juice
½ tsp. garlic powder
1 tsp. minced onion
1 Tbsp. chives, chopped
1 tsp. honey
Celtic Sea Salt, to taste (optional)

Place all ingredients except chives in a blender and blend until smooth. Fold in chives; cover and chill.

One or more of the following can be added: avocado, minced red onion, or diced tomatoes. This is good on baked potatoes. *Serves 6.*

SUSAN WOOD'S SPINACH SALAD DRESSING

1 cup honey
¼ cup minced onion
¼ cup Worcestershire sauce
2 cups olive oil
4 tsp. paprika
1 cup apple cider vinegar

Place all ingredients in blender and blend until smooth. *Serves 6.*

SWEET & SOUR DRESSING

1¼ cups extra-virgin olive oil
1¼ cups raw honey
¾ cup raw apple cider vinegar

Mix well in glass jar. *Serves 6.*

TAHINI DRESSING

2 Tbsp. onion
½ cup fresh lemon juice
1 cup extra-virgin olive oil
⅓ cup tahini
2 garlic cloves
2 Tbsp. pure maple syrup
½ cup water
Celtic Sea Salt, to taste

Place all ingredients in blender and blend until smooth. Chill and serve. *Serves 6.*

TAMARI DRESSING

6 Tbsp. extra-virgin olive oil
1 Tbsp. tamari
1 Tbsp. tahini
½ tsp. honey
2 dashes red wine vinegar
Fresh juice of 1 lemon
Dash of garlic powder

Shake together on glass bowl and serve on salad. *Serves 2.*

TOMATO DRESSING

1 medium-size ripe tomato

½ cup extra-virgin olive oil

¼ cup lemon juice

2 garlic cloves

½ red onion

2 Tbsp. raw honey

Dash hot sauce

Celtic Sea Salt, to taste

Place all ingredients in blender. Blend until smooth. *Serves 4.*

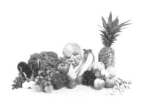

RECIPES FOR DIPS AND SPREADS

BIRCHCREEK SALSA

1 red pepper

1 green pepper

1 small onion

5 large ripe tomatoes, diced

Juice from 2 limes

Fresh cilantro, chopped

Jalapeño peppers, chopped, to taste

Sea salt, to taste

Chop peppers and onion in food processor. Do not overprocess. Mix all ingredients together. Add chopped jalapeños to taste. *Serves 4.*

BLACK BEAN SALSA

2 ears white corn (raw and cut from cob)

1 can black beans, drained and rinsed

½ red pepper, chopped

½ green pepper

½ small sweet onion, chopped

1½ tsp. cumin

1½ tsp. chili powder

Juice from 1 lime

Juice from ½ lemon

1 Tbsp. raw sunflower seeds (optional)

Mix all ingredients together and marinate in refrigerator. *Serves 4.*

||||||||||||||||||||||||||||||||||||||||||||||||||||||||||||||||||||||||||||||||||||||||||||

GUACAMOLE

We've added a few bits and pieces to traditional guacamole. It's fantastic as a dip, sandwich filling, or served on portobello mushrooms and garnished with cucumber slices.

    2 ripe avocados, chopped, then smashed
    3 large tomatoes, chopped small
    1–2 cloves fresh garlic, minced
    ¼ tsp. chili powder (or more if you like it hot)
    Juice of 1 lemon
    1 red pepper, finely diced
    1 green pepper, finely diced
    Sea salt and pepper, to taste (optional)

Combine all ingredients until fairly smooth. *Serves 2.*

||||||||||||||||||||||||||||||||||||||||||||||||||||||||||||||||||||||||||||||||||||||||||||

JULIE'S HUMMUS

    5 cans chickpeas, drained and rinsed
    2 cans black beans, drained and rinsed
    ¼ cup tahini (optional)
    Juice of 2 lemons
    2 dashes tamari
    4 Tbsp. extra-virgin olive oil
    2 garlic cloves (optional)
    Celtic Sea Salt, to taste
    Cumin, to taste (optional)

Blend together in food processor until very smooth. Serve with raw veggies or on a sandwich. *Serves 5.*

|||||||||||||||||||||||||||||||||||||||||||||||||||||||||||||||||||||||||||||||

CHILI LENTILS

½ onion, chopped

4 stalks celery, chopped

3 large carrots, sliced thin

2 Tbsp. extra-virgin olive oil

1 bag lentils

1 Tbsp. chili powder

Dash of tamari

2 plum tomatoes

Dash of balsamic vinegar

Celtic Sea Salt, to taste

Lightly sauté vegetables in oil in large pot. Then, in the same pot with the vegetables, boil the lentils according to package directions. When lentils are tender, stir in chili powder, tamari, tomatoes, vinegar, and salt. Serve with whole-grain bread or roll. *Serves 4.*

|||||||||||||||||||||||||||||||||||||||||||||||||||||||||||||||||||||||||||||||

BABA GHANOUSH

1 medium eggplant

¼ cup lemon juice (or less)

¼ cup tahini

1–2 garlic cloves, chopped

1 tsp. olive oil

Sea salt, to taste (optional)

Fresh parsley, for garnish

Preheat oven to 400 degrees. Pierce the eggplant with a fork a few times and bake for about 40 minutes or until tender and somewhat deflated. Cool, then peel with a fork or knife. Mash the eggplant with a potato masher. Add other ingredients. Serve at room temperature with raw veggies. *Serves 2.*

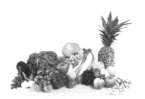

OTHER RECIPES

BROCCOLI RABE

> 2 heads broccoli rabe
> 1 clove elephant garlic, sliced thin (or 2–3 cloves regular garlic)
> Extra-virgin olive oil, enough for sautéing
> Celtic Sea Salt, to taste

Trim to just heads and only thin stems of the broccoli rabe. Rinse.

In a saucepan heat garlic and olive oil until garlic begins to sizzle. Remove from heat. Steam broccoli rabe; cover and allow to wilt slightly. Toss broccoli rabe in oil and garlic and add Celtic Sea Salt to taste.

This is excellent served over whole-wheat pasta. *Serves 2.*

BROCCOLI SUN-DRIED TOMATO SAUTÉ

> ⅛ cup extra-virgin, cold-pressed olive oil
> 1 clove elephant garlic, thinly sliced
> 3 heads broccoli
> ¼ cup sliced almonds
> ½ cup sun-dried tomato, thinly sliced
> Sea salt, to taste

In a saucepan heat olive oil. Add garlic and simmer until garlic begins to sizzle. Remove saucepan from heat.

Trim the entire broccoli head into bite-size pieces, and peel all the main stems with a sharp knife. Slice stems into ⅛- to ¼-inch slices. Steam broccoli until just wilted, about 3 minutes.

Add wilted broccoli, almonds, and sun-dried tomato to saucepan of olive oil and garlic; toss. Add sea salt, to taste. *Serves 2.*

NOTE: To enhance taste, add 2 Tbsp. Worcestershire sauce and ¼ cup water to broccoli and toss—*before* cooking.

CAULIFLOWER "MASHED POTATOES"

1 head cauliflower, cut into small pieces
Dollop of Vegenaise or butter substitute, to taste
Celtic Sea Salt, to taste

Steam cauliflower in a small amount of water until tender. Drain well. Run through food processor with Vegenaise until smooth. Add salt to taste. *Serves 2.*

‖‖‖

SAUTÉED CAULIFLORETS

1 medium head cauliflower
1 garlic clove, crushed
¼ cup extra-virgin olive oil
1½ tsp. dried parsley
1½ tsp. lemon pepper

Break 1 medium head cauliflower into very small bite-size florets to make about 2½ cups. Wash and dry thoroughly. In large pan, sauté the crushed garlic clove in the olive oil. Add the cauliflower and sauté gently for 10–15 minutes, or until tender but still crisp. Drain on paper towel. Add seasonings. Serve warm. *Serves 2.*

‖‖

GREEN POTATOES

3 baking potatoes
2 stalks broccoli
¼ cup Vegenaise (or other vegan mayonnaise substitute)
Splash of almond milk
Celtic Sea Salt, to taste
½ cup rice or soy cheese, shredded

Prick and bake potatoes in moderate oven about 45 minutes or until done. Remove from oven and let cool.

Chop and steam broccoli. Cut potatoes in half the long way and scoop the insides out into a bowl. Add the steamed broccoli, Vegenaise, milk, and sea salt, mashing together (can also be run through food processor).

Spoon mixture into potato skins and arrange on cookie sheet. Sprinkle with shredded rice or soy cheese on each. Warm in oven, about 10–15 minutes. *Serves 3.*

||||||||||||||||||||||||||||||||||||||||||||||||||||||||||||||||||||||||||||||||||||||||||||||||||||

GREEN ZUCCHINI SAUTÉ

3 large green zucchinis
½ tsp. sea salt
1 Tbsp. olive oil for sautéing
1 medium onion, sliced

Shred zucchini in food processor. Toss with ½ tsp. sea salt, and leave in colander for about 15 minutes to drain. Press zucchini to remove remaining liquid. Heat just enough olive oil to sauté onions. Cook onions on medium heat until clear (not brown), about 10 minutes. Add shredded zucchini and continue to cook. Zucchini should be cooked just enough to thoroughly heat, not browned. Serve hot. *Serves 1.*

BIRCHCREEK GRANOLA

    5 cups rolled oats (old fashioned, not instant)
    ½ cup wheat germ (optional)
    ½ cup raw sunflower seeds
    ¼ cup raw sesame seeds
    ½ cup raw pumpkin seeds (pepitas)
    1 cup raw almonds (or walnuts), slivered
    or chopped
    ½–¾ lb. raw, unsweetened dates, chopped
    Organic raisins, to taste (optional)
    Organic dried apricots, to taste (optional)
    1 cup unsweetened coconut (optional)
    ½ cup pure maple syrup
    ½ cup raw honey
    Splash vanilla

In a large bowl combine oats, wheat germ (if using), seeds, almonds, dates, raisins (if using), apricots (if using), and coconut (if using). Mix together well.

Add syrup, honey, and vanilla. Stir until well coated. Spread in thin layers onto lightly oiled cookie sheets and bake in low-temperature oven (275°–300° F) until set. Granola hardens as it cools. *Serves 6.*

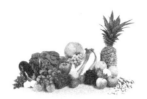

SMOOTHIE RECIPES

FRUIT SMOOTHIES

1 cup frozen fruit (no sugar added) or
fresh fruit
¼ cup rice or almond milk, unsweetened
(optional)
1 Tbsp. raw honey (optional)
Water, just enough for blending

Fill blender or smoothie maker with frozen fruit of your choice, or a combination of fresh and frozen fruit. (If using all fresh fruit, add ice cubes.) Add any combination of the liquids almost to top of fruit. Blend until smooth. *Makes 1 smoothie.*

BIRCHCREEK GREEN SMOOTHIE

1 cup fresh or frozen unsweetened fruit
(mango, peach, pineapple, berries, etc.)
2 Tbsp. raw chia vegetarian protein powder
1 cup raw greens (spinach, kale, mustard
greens, collards, turnip greens, etc.)
½ banana *or* ½ cup unsweetened almond milk
Water to blend

Blend all ingredients in a blender, Vitamix, or smoothie maker until smooth. *Makes 1 smoothie.*

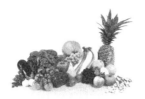

SANDWICH SUGGESTIONS

Breads

Always use a whole-grain or multigrain bread with no processed sugar or preservatives. These will be found in the health food section or freezer section of a good grocery store or health food store. Some examples are: Ezekiel 4:19 bread, Food for Life breads, Alvarado bread, whole-wheat pita bread, and sprouted breads and wraps. In a sandwich, remember that the bread is considered a cooked food, not raw.

Condiments

The best mayonnaise substitute we have found is Vegenaise, located in the refrigerator section of health food stores. Mustard is fine (without mayonnaise or relish added). Ketchup must contain no processed sugar. Consider using one of the fresh salad dressing recipes on your sandwich for a change of taste.

Seasonings

Celtic Sea Salt and black pepper should be used very sparingly. Use no table salt. Consider red-flaked pepper and sesame seeds.

Pickles

You may eat a pickle on the side or several slices in your sandwich for flavor. Read the labels on the pickle jars, and buy only those without added sugar.

Sandwich combinations

The following are only some suggestions among hundreds of possibilities for the sandwich aficionado:

Peanut butter and jelly

This classic can easily be adapted to the Birchcreek program. The ingredients in the peanut butter should be peanuts only, whenever possible. Consider almond butter as a much healthier alternative to peanut butter. Jelly should be fruit only (Smuckers makes one) or apple, pear, or plum butter made with fruit only. Sliced fresh fruit is wonderful on this sandwich. This is not a low-calorie sandwich.

Tofu

Make an eggless salad with lettuce, tomato, and sprouts on multigrain bread. Crumble rinsed tofu and add Vegenaise.

Guacamole

Spread guacamole in whole-wheat pita bread and add shredded lettuce and chopped fresh tomatoes.

Hummus

Easily make your own hummus from our recipe. Then spread in whole-wheat pita bread and add fresh raw baby spinach and sliced red onions.

Baba ghanoush

Make your own from our recipe, and then spread in whole-wheat pita bread. Add thinly sliced cucumbers.

TLT

Add tempeh, lettuce, tomato, and Vegenaise on whole-wheat toast.

Tofu (or tempeh) and sauerkraut

Put baked, marinated tofu (or tempeh) and sauerkraut on sourdough rye, with a pickle on the side.

Tofu and cheese

Melt rice cheese over a baked, breaded tofu cutlet covered with marinara sauce on a whole-wheat baguette.

Avocado

Serve sliced avocado, tomato, lettuce, alfalfa sprouts, and soy or rice cheese on sprouted-wheat bread.

Marinated Vegetable

Put marinated veggies in pita or a wrap.

Raw veggies sandwich

On whole-grain bread layer the following: lettuce, tomato, sliced cucumbers, alfalfa sprouts, sliced olives, sliced red onions, and sliced pickles. Add Vegenaise and balsamic vinegar.

Faux sausage and peppers

Sauté onions and green peppers together. Add a sprinkle of fennel. Serve on a whole-grain hero roll.

Tofu garden salad

Make a sandwich of sliced tofu with lettuce, tomato, sweet relish, and Vegenaise on sprouted-grain bread.

Perry Street Burgers

Add to a vegan veggie burger: sautéed onions, red and green peppers, melted vegan cheese, and marinara sauce on a multi-grain bun.

Santa Fe Burger

Add to a vegan veggie burger: salsa, chopped or mashed avocado, and shredded lettuce on multigrain bun.

Sausalito Burger

Add to a vegan veggie burger: sliced avocado, tomato, lettuce, red onion slices, and Vegenaise on a multigrain bun.

Classic veggie sandwich

Mix sliced tomatoes, cucumbers, green zucchini, and pickles. Place between two large romaine lettuce leaves and sprinkle with shredded carrots. Serve on Ezekiel 4:19 bread spread with mustard and Vegenaise.

Ron's Faux BLT

Layer lettuce, sliced tomato, and baked blue corn chips with sea salt on toasted bread with Vegenaise.

Italian

Place thin-sliced plum tomatoes, rice cheese (mozzarella flavor), and fresh basil leaves, sprinkled with veggie parmesan cheese alternative and drizzled with extra-virgin olive oil—in a whole-grain wrap.

Mexican

Place shredded iceberg lettuce, fresh (see our recipes) or jarred (no sugar) salsa, sliced avocado with fresh (or dried) cilantro leaves on a whole-grain wrap or in a corn taco.

APPENDIX C

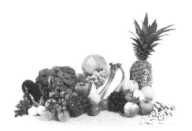

BIRCHCREEK TESTIMONIALS

I'm just back from a one-week juice fast and feel like a new person. I never felt hungry or deprived. The staff tailors the program to fit individual needs. They make you feel pampered and cared for while conducting profound and valuable workshops on nutrition and weight loss. I received lots of good tips about how to make permanent lifestyle changes. Glorious location—didn't want to leave and can't wait to go back.

—D.C.

The reward after spending a week of cleansing the body, mind, and spirit is that you feel wonderful. Your mind is clear, your skin feels soft, and your digestion is free of the many toxins you become overloaded with despite eating well and taking decent care of yourself. You will feel and look amazing, and the benefit is that you will perhaps take home some of the valuable and insightful information Ron and Julie share and make changes to your eating habits and lifestyle that will stay with you in the long run.

The juice fasting program that Ron and Julie have developed over the past ten years is thorough, beneficial, and effective. Their juices taste wonderful and are packed with nutrition. They are also easy to replicate at home should you wish to continue incorporating healthy juices into your diet. Expect to take in a lot of information and make healthy and life-changing alterations to your diet and wellness. After all, we all want to feel and look our best, and the Birchcreek Retreat can give you a jump start to achieving a more healthful lifestyle.

—E.D.

I lost eight pounds my first week. My skin was tingling, I had so much energy, I slept like a baby and woke up with no problem, my thoughts and memory were crystal clear, and I felt ten years younger (I'm thirty-three). Before that I was fat, lazy, lethargic, out of shape, and totally unmotivated. I also ate around the clock and was still always hungry. What a difference!

—G.F.

The most pleasant surprise for me was how much I learned about our bodies and digestive system through Ron's daily seminars. He completely opened my eyes. But they don't just tell you what NOT to eat. They show you how to eat properly, and Julie did several workshops on how to make a healthy sandwich, order food at a restaurant, prepare pasta, etc. You also leave with a pile of recipes. They even teach you what to look for when reading food labels. I will never grocery shop the same way again.

—K.J.

I spent just four days at Birchcreek and I am very relaxed. I feel great, and I lost 8.5 pounds.

—MAEN AJLYAKIN

It has been two weeks since I left Birchcreek, and I want to thank the entire staff for a truly life-changing, priceless experience. I have spent thousands of dollars on diets, diet pills, diet books—you name it....Your program should be mandatory for everyone. I see a light at the end of the tunnel, and it is not a train wreck! I will be back soon. Accept my deep thanks and appreciation to all at Birchcreek.

—C.B.

The benefits I derived from my stay at Birchcreek are astounding. I came because I had difficulty losing weight on my own and needed help. Since adopting your program, in addition to losing weight, I have rid myself of arthritis, lost my susceptibility to allergies, and cured my occasional bouts with psoriasis. You set me on a new and correct path to follow for the rest of my life, and for that I am truly indebted.

—BILL KAPLAN

I participated in the Weekend Warrior, and it was awesome! The Birchcreek staff was professional, informative, and supportive. I was able to refocus my weight-loss efforts and lost five pounds in two days. Thank you for a great weekend!

—O.N.

My four-week stay at Birchcreek changed the way I look at, think about, and feel about food. I enjoyed everything from Ron's seminars, which bombard you with facts about nutrition and the importance of eating right, to Elizabeth's lectures where I learned that food is not something you fear but something to enjoy. Thanks so much!

—N.S.

Excellent place to do a juice fast, lose weight, and gain a new perspective. You enter a home when you go to Birchcreek, and they take care of you like a family member. It is always encouraging, but there's plenty of space and privacy.

—N.B.

My experience at Birchcreek was absolutely incredible. Birchcreek is first and foremost a diet/detox center located just off the main road on a beautiful wooded property right next to a stream. While the aged facility is pretty typical for the Catskills, the program is not. In fact, the program is not typical at all. Let me explain.

As it happened, I had blood work done before I came to Birchcreek. I decided to have the same blood work done after I returned home from the month-long program there.

In one month I lost thirty-four pounds, reduced my cholesterol thirty-two points, reduced my triglycerides by forty-two points, and reduced my glucose by twenty points...just to name a few results. And for all you who are part of the "protein police" and maintain that you "need" meat protein, my levels of protein were only slightly lower than they were when I began. All this while eating a plant-based diet and juicing fruits and vegetables.

The program at Birchcreek is effective because it is something anyone can do... and they teach you how to do it. The seminars deal with the why, and the cooking and education classes deal with the how. The meals and the total experience deal with the fact that if you will do it, it works. It is that simple.

In the first two lectures I received an explanation of what I have been experiencing for years. It was why I found weight loss so difficult. Not one doctor, dietician, or nutritionist had ever given me anything but the standard "you simply have to burn more calories than you take in" mantra. Eat the standard American diet in smaller portions, and you will lose weight. I'm sorry, but some of us don't. Something is going on in our bodies for which we have no control that shuts that process down, as the autonomic system tries desperately to keep up with the stressed biology in the body.

In my case, it took almost the full four weeks to reset my metabolic system. After coming home, I have continued on the program and have continued to drop additional weight. This is good, because I have additional weight to lose.

In conclusion, if you are tired of going around in circles with your diet and want a comprehensive program that really works, then Birchcreek could be for you. You will find that the staff is excellent, professional, and personable, and they approach each person's situation individually.

—P.M.

Yes, I lost ten pounds from the juice fast, but that wasn't the true value of my week there. I came away with the tools, knowledge, and commitment to keep my new healthy lifestyle going forward. The directors of the program and their caring staff are very invested in each guest and their individual success. Their favorite question, "How's that working for you?", leads you to pause and reflect on your current eating/ exercise habits, and in my case, the answer was: "They're not working for me at all!" But they are now…thanks to Birchcreek. I would wholeheartedly recommend Birchcreek to anyone stuck in a rut and looking to make a healthy change. Having seven days away from everyday temptations and routines and being immersed in a peaceful, nurturing, nutritious, and physically active environment in the middle of the woods was the best thing I have ever done for myself!

—R.S.

When I arrived at Birchcreek, I was in very poor health. I was suffering from fibromyalgia-type symptoms along with many hormone-related issues that were altering my ability to function on a daily basis. I was going to begin taking a prescribed medication for my symptoms but decided to wait until I returned from Birchcreek. After the fifth day on the juice fast I realized that *all* of my symptoms were gone! I had no pain in my body, I was thinking more clearly, and my hot flashes were gone. I had more energy than I have had in a long time. The juice fast results were amazing! After returning home I have continued to walk as part of my daily routine and have added a mile to my walk. I lost seven pounds during my ten-day stay at the retreat and an additional eight pounds since I've been home.

—J.R.

My wife, Suzanne, wound up in the intensive care unit with one of the highest diabetic blood sugar levels (1951) ever recorded at Bassett Hospital in Coopertown, New York. The doctor's prognosis for my wife's type 2 diabetic condition was a lifetime of ever-increasing medication and a diet, which confused and depressed us both. That motivated us to seek knowledge and alternative means to cope with her condition.

Both my wife and I had considerable weight to lose. We found the Birchcreek program, which boasted of remarkable results for type 2 diabetics. Suzanne decided to attend for one month, and I agreed to attend as a show of support. We did, and within two weeks her numbers had dropped dramatically. Her doctor began, somewhat reluctantly, to reduce her insulin each week. That trend continued every week, and within six weeks Suzanne was completely off medication and with normal blood sugar levels. Within four months she lost seventy pounds, I lost sixty pounds, and we both felt better than we had in years.

Today, five years after our visit to Birchcreek, my wife remains healthy and free of any diabetic symptoms, and we have both adopted the Birchcreek eating plan as our own.

—Ed Rivera

NOTES

CHAPTER 4
A VERY SAD DIET

1. Centers for Disease Control and Prevention, "Smoking and Tobacco Use—Highlights: Warning Labels," http://www.cdc.gov/tobacco/data_statistics/sgr/2000/highlights/labels/index.htm (accessed January 18, 2012).

2. *The Miraculous Self-Healing Body,* hosted by George Malkmus (Shelby, NC: Hallelujah Acres, 2007), DVD series.

3. S. Jay Olshansky et al., "A Potential Decline in Life Expectancy in the United States in the 21st Century," *New England Journal of Medicine* 352 (March 2005): 1138–1145, http://www.nejm.org/doi/full/10.1056/NEJMsr043743#t=articleTop (accessed January 18, 2012).

CHAPTER 5
ADJUSTING YOUR FRAME OF REFERENCE

1. *The Week*, "Briefing: The Childhood Obesity Epidemic," October 25, 2007, http://theweek.com/article/index/27720/briefing_the_child-hood_obesity_epidemic (accessed January 18, 2012).

2. Ibid.

3. Ibid.

4. Olshansky et al., "A Potential Decline in Life Expectancy in the United States in the 21st Century."

5. National Institutes of Health, "Obesity Threatens to Cut U.S. Life Expectancy, New Analysis Suggests," *NIH News*, news release, March 16, 2005, http://www.nih.gov/news/pr/mar2005/nia-16.htm (accessed January 18, 2012).

6. T. Colin Campbell and Thomas M. Campbell II, *The China Study* (Dallas: BenBella Books, 2006), 2.

CHAPTER 7
YOUR ENZYME BANK ACCOUNT—THE WEAK LINK

1. Allison Chilcott, "Are California's Children Physically Fit?," *Growing Up Well*, http://www.chipolicy.org/pdf/PhysFit.pdf (accessed February 7, 2012).

2. Edward Howell, *Enzyme Nutrition* (New York: Avery/Penguin Putnam, 1985), 5.

CHAPTER 8
CHARTING A NEW COURSE

1. "The Wrong Fuel," *The Miraculous Self-Healing Body.*

2. Ibid.

3. Barbara Starfield, "Is US Health Really the Best in the World?", *Journal of the American Medical Association* 284, no. 4 (July 26, 2000): 483–485.

4. Kathy Freston, "There Is a Way to Help Avoid Heart Disease and Diabetes: You Are What You Eat!", Alternet.org, October 31, 2009, http://www.alternet.org/health/143633?page=entire (accessed January 18, 2012).

CHAPTER 11
DON'T PHOOL WITH YOUR PH

1. The-Sleep-Zone.com, "Sleep Deprivation Symptoms," http://www.the-sleep-zone.com/sleep-deprivation-symptoms.html (accessed January 20, 2012).

2. Food and Drug Administration, "Labeling Guidance for Estrogen Drug Products, Physician Labeling, Revised August 1992," http://www.fda.gov/ohrms/dockets/ac/99/backgrd/3557b1e.pdf (accessed January 20, 2012).

3. Michael Castleman, "The Calcium Myth," AlternativeMedicine.com, http://www.alternativemedicine.com/calcium/calcium-myth (accessed January 20, 2012).

4. Ibid.

5. Ibid.

6. Ibid.

CHAPTER 12
EXCITOTOXINS

1. Russell L. Blaylock, *Excitotoxins: The Taste That Kills* (Santa Fe, NM: Health Press, 1996).

2. Barbara L. Minton, "Red Clover Blocks Neurological Damage From MSG," NaturalNews.com, September 22, 2008, http://www.naturalnews.com/024275.html (accessed January 20, 2012).

3. More information can be found at http://www.russellblaylockmd.com and http://dorway.com/.

4. Paul Fassa, "Protect Yourself From MSG and Aspartame Excitotoxicity," NaturalNews.com, May 7, 2009, http://www.naturalnews.com/026216_MSG_aspartame_excitotoxin.html (accessed January 23, 2012).

CHAPTER 13
HEREDITY: IT'S MY PARENTS' FAULT

1. ScienceDaily.com, "Obesity Increases Cancer Risk, Analysis of Hundreds of Studies Shows," February 17, 2008, http://www.sciencedaily.com/releases/2008/02/080217211802.htm (accessed January 23, 2012).

2. ScienceDaily.com, "Strong Link Between Obesity and Colorectal Cancer," December 14, 2007, http://www .sciencedaily.com/releases/2007/12/071214094112.htm (accessed January 23, 2012).

3. American Cancer Society, "Cancer Facts and Figures 2011," http://www.cancer.org/acs/groups/content/@ epidemiologysurveilance/documents/document/acspc-029771 .pdf (accessed January 23, 2012).

4. National Cancer Institute, "BRCA1 and BRCA2: Cancer Risk and Genetic Testing," fact sheet, May 29, 2009, http://www .cancer.gov/cancertopics/factsheet/Risk/BRCA (accessed January 23, 2012).

5. John Herring, "Beating Cancer: Does Early Detection Help?" (blog), Complementary and Alternative Medicine Community, November 5, 2009, http://www.wellsphere.com/ complementary-alternative-medicine-article/beating-cancer -does-early-detection-help/870011 (accessed January 23, 2012). "Report to the Nation: Cancer Death Rates Drop, but Total Number of Cases Rise," *CA: A Cancer Journal for Clinicians* 52, no. 4 (July/August 2002): 186–188, http://onlinelibrary.wiley .com/doi/10.3322/canjclin.52.4.186/full (accessed January 23, 2012). See also these reports from other sources about other diseases: Agency for Healthcare Research and Quality, "Osteoporosis-Linked Fractures Rise Dramatically," *AHRQ News and Numbers*, July 17, 2009, http://www.ahrq.gov/news/ nn/nn071709.htm (accessed January 23, 2012). University of Chicago, "Diabetes Cases to Double and Costs to Triple by 2034," *UChicago News*, November 27, 2009, http://news .uchicago.edu/article/2009/11/27/diabetes-cases-double-and -costs-triple-2034 (accessed January 23, 2012). Medical News Today, "Heart Disease May Be on the Rise According to Mayo Clinic Population Research," February 12, 2008, http://www .medicalnewstoday.com/releases/96989.php (accessed January 23, 2012).

CHAPTER 15
INTERCEPTING THE TIPPING POINT

1. Christianna Pierce, compiler, "List of Anti-Angiogenic Foods," *Elegant Simple Life* (blog), May 25, 2010, http://www .elegantsimplelife.com/2010/05/list-of-anti-angiogenic-foods/ (accessed January 23, 2012). Copyright © 2010. Used with permission of Christianna Pierce.

CHAPTER 16
THE PROTEIN GAP

1. Robynne Boyd, "Weight Is Key to Protein Requirements," WebMD.com, November 7, 2008, http://www.webmd.com/ food-recipes/news/20081107/weight-is-key-to-protein -requirements (accessed January 23, 2012). Simplebean.com, "Protein/Weight Ratio," http://www.simplebean.com/hg/pwr .aspx (accessed January 23, 2012).

2. T. Colin Campbell and Thomas M. Campbell II, *The China Study* (Dallas: BenBella Books, 2006).

CHAPTER 17
WORKING TOGETHER

1. Francis Marion Pottenger Jr., *Pottenger's Cats: A Study in Nutrition* (Lemon Grove, CA: Price-Pottenger Nutrition Foundation, Inc., 1983, 1995).

2. "The Anti-Aging Diet," Raw Food Health, http://www.raw -food-health.net/Anti-Aging-Diet.html (accessed February 6, 2012).

3. For more information, visit Dr. Barnard's website at http:// www.nealbarnard.org (accessed January 24, 2012).

4. As quoted in "Beat Heart Disease With a Vegan Diet," *Gobble Green* (blog), August 10, 2009, http://gobblegreen.com/ blog/?m=200908 (accessed January 24, 2012).

5. For more information, visit Dr. Fuhrman's website at http:// www.drfuhrman.com (accessed January 24, 2012).

6. For more information, visit Dr. McDougall's website at http://www.drmcdougall.com (accessed January 24, 2012).

7. For more information, visit Dr. Blaylock's website at http://www.blaylockreport.com (accessed January 24, 2012).

8. For more information, visit Dr. Campbell's website at http://www.tcolincampbell.org/courses-resources/home (accessed January 24, 2012).

9. For more information, visit Dr. Young's website at http://www.phmiracleliving.com (accessed January 24, 2012).

10. Liz Cho, "What's in Your Money-Saving Multivitamins?", WABC TV, August 13, 2010, http://abclocal.go.com/wabc/story?section=news/consumer&id=7607655 (accessed January 24, 2012).

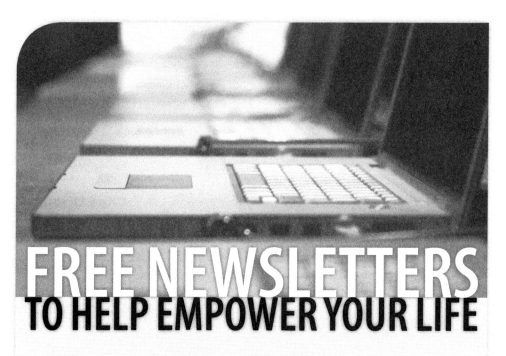